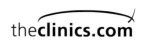

HEMATOLOGY/ ONCOLOGY CLINICS OF NORTH AMERICA

Antiphospholipid Thrombosis Syndromes

GUEST EDITORS
Rodger L. Bick, MD, PhD, FACP
and William F. Baker, Jr, MD, FACP

February 2008 • Volume 22 • Number 1

SAUNDERS

An Imprint of Elsevier, Inc.
PHILADELPHIA   LONDON   TORONTO   MONTREAL   SYDNEY   TOKYO

W.B. SAUNDERS COMPANY
A Division of Elsevier Inc.

Elsevier Inc. • 1600 John F. Kennedy Boulevard • Suite 1800 • Philadelphia, Pennsylvania 19103-2899

http://www.hemonc.theclinics.com

HEMATOLOGY/ONCOLOGY CLINICS OF NORTH AMERICA February 2008 Editor: Kerry Holland	Volume 22, Number 1 ISSN 0889-8588 ISBN-13: 978-1-4160-5842-7 ISBN-10: 1-4160-5842-7

Copyright © 2008 by Elsevier Inc. All rights reserved. No part of this publication may be reproduced or transmitted in any form or by any means, electronic or mechanical, including photocopy, recording, or any information retrieval system, without written permission from the publisher.

Single photocopies of single articles may be made for personal use as allowed by national copyright laws. Permission of the publisher and payment of a fee is required for all other photocopying, including multiple or systematic copying, copying for advertising or promotional purposes, resale, and all forms of document delivery. Special rates are available for educational institutions that wish to make photocopies for non-profit educational classroom use. Permission may be sought directly from Elsevier's Global Rights Department in Oxford, UK: Phone: 215-239-3804 or +44 (0)1865 843830; Fax: +44 (0)1865 853333; E-mail: healthpermissions@elsevier.com. Requests may also be completed online via the Elsevier homepage (http://www.elsevier.com/permissions). In the USA, users may clear permissions and make payments through the Copyright Clearance Center, Inc., 222 Rosewood Drive, Danvers, MA 01923, USA; Phone: (978) 750-8400, Fax: (978) 750-4744, and in the UK through the Copyright Licensing Agency Rapid Clearance Service (CLARCS), 90 Tottenham Court Road, London W1P 0LP, UK; Phone: (+44) 171 436 5931; Fax: (+44) 171 436 3986. Others countries may have a local reprographic rights agency for payments.

Reprints: For copies of 100 or more, of articles in this publication, please contact the Commercial Reprints Department, Elsevier Inc., 360 Park Avenue South, New York, New York 10010-1710. Tel. (212) 633-3813; Fax: (212) 462-1935; E-mail: reprints@elsevier.com.

The ideas and opinions expressed in *Hematology/Oncology Clinics of North America* do not necessarily reflect those of the Publisher. The Publisher does not assume any responsibility for any injury and/or damage to persons or property arising out of or related to any use of the material contained in this periodical. The reader is advised to check the appropriate medical literature and the product information currently provided by the manufacturer of each drug to be administered to verify the dosage, the method and duration of administration, or contraindications. It is the responsibility of the treating physician or other health care professional, relying on independent experience and knowledge of the patient, to determine drug dosages and the best treatment of the patient. Mention of any product in this issue should not be construed as endorsement by the contributors, editors, or the Publisher of the product or manufacturers' claims.

Hematology/Oncology Clinics (ISSN 0889-8588) is published bimonthly by Elsevier Inc., 360 Park Avenue South, New York, NY 10010-1710. Months of issue are February, April, June, August, October, and December. Business and Editorial Offices: 1600 John F. Kennedy Blvd., Suite 1800, Philadelphia, PA 19103-2899. Customer Service Office: 6277 Sea Harbor Drive, Orlando, FL 32887-4800. Periodicals postage paid at New York, NY and additional mailing offices. Subscription prices are $262.00 per year (US individuals), $392.00 per year (US institutions), $131.00 per year (US students), $297.00 per year (Canadian individuals), $470.00 per year (Canadian institutions), $166.00 per year (Canadian students), $332.00 per year (international individuals), $470.00 per year (international institutions), $166.00 per year (international students). International air speed delivery is included in all *Clinics* subscription prices. All prices are subject to change without notice. **POSTMASTER:** Send address changes to *Hematology/Oncology Clinics of North America*, Elsevier Periodicals Customer Service, 6277 Sea Harbor Drive, Orlando, FL 32887-4800. Customer Service: 1-800-654-2452 (US). From outside of the US, call 1-407-345-4000.

Hematology/Oncology Clinics of North America is covered in *Index Medicus*, *EMBASE/Excerpta Medica*, and *BIOSIS*.

Printed in the United States of America.

HEMATOLOGY/ONCOLOGY CLINICS OF NORTH AMERICA

Antiphospholipid Thrombosis Syndromes

GUEST EDITORS

RODGER L. BICK, MD, PhD, FACP, Retired Clinical Professor of Medicine and Pathology, University of Texas Southwestern Medical Center, Dallas, Texas

WILLIAM F. BAKER, Jr, MD, FACP, Associate Clinical Professor, David Geffen School of Medicine, Center for Health Sciences, University of California, Los Angeles; Director, Thrombosis, Hemostasis and Special Hematology Clinic, Kern Medical Center; California Clinical Thrombosis Center, Bakersfield, California

CONTRIBUTORS

CAFAR ADIGUZEL, MD, Department of Pathology, Loyola University Chicago, Maywood, Illinois

NAVIN M. AMIN, MD, DTM&H, Associate Professor of Medicine, David Geffen School of Medicine, University of California, Los Angeles; Professor of Family Medicine, University of California Irvine Medical Center, Orange; Associate Professor of Family Medicine, Stanford University, Stanford; Chairman, Department of Family Medicine, Kern Medical Center, Bakersfield, California

WILLIAM F. BAKER, Jr, MD, FACP, Associate Clinical Professor, David Geffen School of Medicine, Center for Health Sciences, University of California, Los Angeles; Director, Thrombosis, Hemostasis and Special Hematology Clinic, Kern Medical Center; California Clinical Thrombosis Center, Bakersfield, California

RODGER L. BICK, MD, PhD, FACP, Retired Clinical Professor of Medicine and Pathology, University of Texas Southwestern Medical Center, Dallas, Texas

JOSÉ BILLER, MD, FACP, FAAN, FAHA, Professor of Neurology and Neurological Surgery; and Chairman, Department of Neurology, Loyola University Chicago, Stritch School of Medicine, Maywood, Illinois

RIMA M. DAFER, MD, MPH, FAHA, Associate Professor of Neurology and Neurological Surgery, Department of Neurology, Loyola University Chicago, Stritch School of Medicine, Maywood, Illinois

NANCY FABBRINI, MT(ASCP), Department of Pathology, Edward Hines VA Hospital, Hines, Illinois

CONTRIBUTORS continued

JAWED FAREED, PhD, FAHA, Professor, Department of Pathology and Pharmacology; and Professor, Department of Cardiovascular Surgery, Loyola University Chicago, Maywood, Illinois

DEBRA A. HOPPENSTEADT, PhD, SH, MT(ASCP), Associate Professor, Department of Pathology, Stritch School of Medicine, Loyola University Chicago, Maywood, Illinois

FERDINAND LEYA, MD, Professor of Medicine, and Director, Cardiac Catheterization Laboratory, Loyola University Medical Center, Maywood, Illinois

BRIAN R. LONG, MD, Tennessee Heart & Vascular Institute, P.C., Skyline Medical Center, Nashville, Tennessee

HARRY L. MESSMORE, MD, Department of Pathology, Loyola University Chicago, Maywood, Illinois

ROCHELLA A. OSTROWSKI, MD, Fellow in Rheumatology, Division of Rheumatology, Department of Medicine, Loyola University Medical Center, Maywood, Illinois

CHI PHAM, MD, Fellow, The University of Texas Southwestern Medical Center at Dallas, Dallas, Texas

WARREN PIETTE, MD, Chairman, Division of Dermatology, John H. Stroger, Jr. Hospital of Cook County; Professor, Department of Dermatology, Rush University Medical Center, Chicago, Illinois

JOHN A. ROBINSON, MD, Professor of Medicine and Microbiology, Division of Rheumatology, Department of Medicine, Loyola University Medical Center, Maywood, Illinois

YU-MIN SHEN, MD, Assistant Professor, The University of Texas Southwestern Medical Center at Dallas, Dallas, Texas

JEANINE M. WALENGA, PhD, Professor, Thoracic and Cardiovascular Surgery and Pathology, Stritch School of Medicine, Cardiovascular Institute, Loyola University Chicago, Maywood, Illinois

SARI WEINSTEIN, MD, Chief Resident, Division of Dermatology, John H. Stroger, Jr. Hospital of Cook County, Chicago, Illinois

HEMATOLOGY/ONCOLOGY CLINICS OF NORTH AMERICA

Antiphospholipid Thrombosis Syndromes

CONTENTS   VOLUME 22 • NUMBER 1 • FEBRUARY 2008

Dedication   xi

Preface   xiii
Rodger L. Bick and William F. Baker, Jr

The Relationship Between the Antiphospholipid Syndrome and Heparin-Induced Thrombocytopenia   1
Debra A. Hoppensteadt and Jeanine M. Walenga

> Antiphospholipid syndrome (APS) and heparin-induced thrombocytopenia (HIT) are immune-mediated thrombotic conditions caused by antibodies targeted to a protein-antigen complex. Although each disorder is attributed to two distinct antibodies, these autoimmune disorders are characterized by a similar pathogenesis that includes a hypercoagulable state, platelet activation, damage to the vascular endothelium, and inflammation. APS and HIT share similarities in the clinical presentation because each is associated with thrombocytopenia, a high risk of thrombosis in all venous and arterial sites, and catastrophic thrombotic outcomes occur if untreated. Understanding the disease process for one disorder could potentially aid in understanding the other disorder.

Laboratory Evaluation of the Antiphospholipid Syndrome   19
Debra A. Hoppensteadt, Nancy Fabbrini, Rodger L. Bick, Harry L. Messmore, Cafar Adiguzel, and Jawed Fareed

> Antiphospholipid syndrome (APLS) is among the most common acquired blood protein defects that have been identified as leading to thrombosis. This article describes the laboratory diagnosis of APLS, including the detection of lupus anticoagulants, anticardiolipin antibodies, and subtypes of antiphospholipid antibodies.

The Clinical Spectrum of Antiphospholipid Syndrome   33
William F. Baker, Jr and Rodger L. Bick

> Antiphospholipid syndrome (APS) is a disorder characterized by a wide variety of clinical manifestations. Virtually any organ system or tissue may be affected by the consequences of large- or small-vessel thrombosis. There is a broad spectrum of disease among individuals with antiphospholipid antibodies (aPL). Patients may exhibit clinical features suggesting APS but not fulfill the International Criteria for a "definite"

diagnosis. Seronegative APS patients demonstrate typical idiopathic thromboses but aPL are not initially detected. Patients defined with definite APS demonstrate nearly identical sites of venous and arterial thrombosis, regardless of the presence or absence of systemic lupus erythematosus. Microangiopathic APS may present with isolated tissue and organ injury or as the overwhelming "thrombotic storm" observed in catastrophic APS.

Antiphospholipid Antibody Syndrome and Autoimmune Diseases 53
Rochella A. Ostrowski and John A. Robinson

The arbitrary division between antiphospholipid antibody syndrome and secondary antiphospholipid antibody syndrome has not proven useful. Antiphospholipid antibodies in the absence of antiphospholipid antibody syndrome often occur as epiphenomena in many autoimmune diseases. They are very common in systemic lupus erythematosus. Antiphospholipid antibody syndrome is a significant comorbidity in lupus but is uncommon in Sjögren's syndrome, rheumatoid arthritis, scleroderma, and systemic vasculitis. Evidence is growing that antiphospholipid antibodies may have a pathogenic role in pulmonary hypertension and accelerated atherosclerosis of autoimmune diseases.

Cutaneous Manifestations of Antiphospholipid Antibody Syndrome 67
Sari Weinstein and Warren Piette

Many different cutaneous lesions or cutaneous-systemic syndromes can be the presenting sign of antiphospholipid antibody syndrome (APS), or can develop during the course of disease. None of these conditions are specific for APS. Livedo reticularis or racemosa is commonly seen in APS, but it is one of the least specific findings. Other diseases are less commonly seen, in either their idiopathic or APS-associated form, but are more suggestive of APS. APS should be considered in patients who may appear to have idiopathic livedo reticularis with cerebrovascular accidents (Sneddon's syndrome), atrophie blanche, livedoid vasculitis, malignant atrophic papulosis, or anetoderma. Finally, retiform (branching, stellate) purpura or necrosis is perhaps the most characteristic cutaneous lesion of many different cutaneous microvascular occlusion syndromes, including APS.

The Role of Antiphospholipid Syndrome in Cardiovascular Disease 79
Brian R. Long and Ferdinand Leya

The antiphospholipid syndrome (APS) is associated with various cardiovascular manifestations. These include accelerated atherosclerosis, valvular heart disease, intracardiac thrombi, myocardial and pericardial involvement, cerebral and peripheral vascular disease, and premature restenosis of vein grafts and coronary stents. This article reviews the prevalence and proposed mechanisms of the various cardiovascular diseases associated with APS. It concludes with a discussion of current recommendations for treatment of these conditions.

Antiphospholipid Syndrome: Role of Antiphospholipid Antibodies in Neurology 95
Rima M. Dafer and José Biller

Antiphospholipid antibodies (aPLs) are acquired antibodies against anionic phospholipid containing moieties in cell membranes. Their presence often is associated with the antiphospholipid syndrome (APS), an acquired autoimmune prothrombotic syndrome associated with thrombosis in the arterial and venous circulations, recurrent unexplained fetal loss, and thrombocytopenia. The association of aPLs with other nonthrombotic neurological disorders remains of unclear significance. This article reviews the definition of APS, its clinical presentations, and therapeutic approaches.

Antiphospholipid Syndrome in Pregnancy 107
Rodger L. Bick

During the past 5 years the author and his colleagues have assessed carefully 351 women referred for evaluation of thrombosis and hemostasis after they had suffered recurrent miscarriages. This article describes the flow protocol the author and associates follow to maximize success and keep the costs of evaluation of recurrent miscarriage syndrome/infertility at a minimum while providing the best chances for defining a cause and thus providing optimal therapy for successful term pregnancy outcome. It presents the outcomes of the author's protocol and those of others in treating women who have antiphospholipid syndrome and who have suffered recurrent miscarriages.

Antiphospholipid Antibodies and Malignancy 121
Chi Pham and Yu-Min Shen

Antiphospholipid antibody syndrome is characterized clinically by venous or arterial thrombosis, recurrent fetal loss, or placental insufficiency in women. This article describes the prevalence of malignancy, the manifestations, and the prognosis for this condition.

Antiphospholipid Syndromes in Infectious Diseases 131
Navin M. Amin

Antiphospholipid antibodies are essential in the diagnosis of antiphospholipid syndrome (APS), or the classic "Hughes syndrome," which is a systemic disorder that is autoimmune in nature. They are also found in various infections in low titers without any evidence of thrombotic manifestations of APS. However, in a few infections, when antiphospholipid antibodies are associated with protein cofactor, there can be associated thrombosis. Different infections are also responsible for triggering a subset of lethal APS, acute catastrophic APS. This situation requires prompt diagnosis and aggressive treatment of the infection to prevent severe complications.

Treatment Options for Patients Who Have Antiphospholipid Syndromes   145
Rodger L. Bick and William F. Baker, Jr

> The antiphospholipid thrombosis syndrome, associated with anticardiolipin (aCL) or subgroup antibodies, can be divided into one of six subgroups (I–VI). There is little overlap (about 10% or less) between these subtypes, and patients usually conveniently fit into only one of these clinical types. Although there appears to be no correlation with the type, or titer, of aCL antibody and type of syndrome, the subclassification of thrombosis and aCL antibody patients into these groups is important from the therapy standpoint. This article also reviews the clinical presentations associated with each of these six subgroups.

Controversies and Unresolved Issues in Antiphospholipid Syndrome Pathogenesis and Management   155
William F. Baker, Jr, Rodger L. Bick, and Jawed Fareed

> While much is understood concerning the clinical features of patients with antiphospholipid syndrome (APS), many issues remain. The proper designation of patients with "definite" APS and the correct categorization of patients by both laboratory and clinical features are matters of ongoing debate. Recent proposals have identified new subsets of patients who have many typical features of APS but either do not fit the criteria for a "definite" diagnosis or have initially negative laboratory tests for antiphospholipid antibodies. Meanwhile, decisions about laboratory tests are based on expert opinion, rather than the results of controlled trials. As for treatment, many guidelines are offered, but few are backed by data from strong clinical trials. This article summarizes the clinical questions remaining to be answered and debates concerning pathogenesis, diagnosis, and management.

Index   175

HEMATOLOGY/ONCOLOGY CLINICS OF NORTH AMERICA

FORTHCOMING ISSUES

April 2008
Cancer Survivorship
Lois B. Travis, MD and Joachim Yahalom, MD
Guest Editors

June 2008
Thymoma and Thymic Carcinoma
Cesar Moran, MD
Guest Editor

August 2008
Integrative Medicine in Oncology
Moshe Frenkel, MD and Jonathan Cohen, MD
Guest Editors

RECENT ISSUES

December 2007
Multiple Myeloma
Kenneth C. Anderson, MD
Guest Editor

October 2007
Hodgkin's Lymphoma: New Insights in an Old Disease
Volker Diehl, MD, Andreas Engert, MD, and Daniel Re, MD
Guest Editors

August 2007
Platelet Disorders
Ravindra Sarode, MD
Guest Editor

THE CLINICS ARE NOW AVAILABLE ONLINE!

Access your subscription at:
http://www.theclinics.com

Dedication

Dr. Rodger Bick and Dr. William Baker dedicate this issue of *Hematology/Oncology Clinics of North America* to their wives: Marilyn Bick and Sharon Baker.

Preface

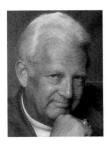 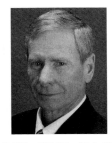

Rodger L. Bick, MD, PhD, FACP
William F. Baker, Jr, MD, FACP
Guest Editors

This issue of *Hematology Oncology Clinics of North America* is dedicated to the topic of antiphospholipid syndromes. The antiphospholipid syndromes are the most common of the acquired thrombophilias but remain unclear and confusing to most clinicians and physicians in general. These disorders commonly lead to arterial and venous thrombosis and other serious clinical sequelae, but many physicians forget to consider testing for antiphospholipid syndrome when faced with these events. Indeed, many do not recognize the different antiphospholipid antibodies that may be associated with these events. These antibodies include lupus anticoagulants, anticardiolipin antibodies, beta-2-glycoprotein-1, and antiphospholipid antibody subgroups including antiphosphatidylserine, antiphosphatidylinositol, antiphosphatidylcholine, antiphosphatidylglycerol, antiphosphatidylethanolamine, antiphosphatidic acid, antiannexin-V, and hexagonal phospholipids. These antiphospholipid antibodies lead to thrombotic, thromboembolic, and other catastrophic events in a wide variety of medical and surgical settings. Thus this issue is written by experts in the various specialties in which antiphospholipid syndromes are most commonly seen. In addition sections are dedicated to laboratory diagnostic features and available tests, pathophysiology, and controversies.

We hope this issue will increase awareness and appreciation for these serious syndromes and thus result in rapid diagnosis and treatment and better patient care.

Rodger L. Bick, MD, PhD, FACP
10455 North Central Expressway, Suite 109-320
Dallas, TX 75231, USA

E-mail address: rbick@thrombosis.com

William F. Baker, Jr, MD, FACP
David Geffen School of Medicine
Center for Health Sciences
University of California, Los Angeles
Los Angeles, CA, USA

Thrombosis, Hemostasis and Special Hematology Clinic
Kern Medical Center
Bakersfield, CA 93311, USA

California Clinical Thrombosis Center
9330 Stockdale Highway, Suite 300
Bakersfield, CA 93311, USA

E-mail address: wbaker@thrombosiscenter.com

HEMATOLOGY/ONCOLOGY CLINICS OF NORTH AMERICA

The Relationship Between the Antiphospholipid Syndrome and Heparin-Induced Thrombocytopenia

Debra A. Hoppensteadt, PhD, SH, MT(ASCP)[a],
Jeanine M. Walenga, PhD[b],*

[a]Department of Pathology, Stritch School of Medicine, Loyola University Chicago, 2160 S. First Avenue, Maywood, IL 60153, USA
[b]Stritch School of Medicine, Cardiovascular Institute, Building 110, Room 5226, Loyola University Chicago, 2160 S. First Avenue, Maywood, IL 60153, USA

Patients recognized to be at increased risk for thrombosis have been referred to as having a hypercoagulable state or thrombophilia. There are two disorders that are characterized by unexplained thrombosis in the presence of specific antibodies: the antiphospholipid syndrome (APS), and heparin-induced thrombocytopenia (HIT). Both disorders are defined as having a hypercoagulable state associated with antibody-mediated thrombosis.

Although caused by two distinct antibodies, it has been suggested that HIT and APS are similar in terms of an autoimmune pathophysiologic mechanism [1,2]. Both HIT and APS are caused by antibodies, targeted to a protein-antigen complex, which bind to FcγIIa receptors. The antibodies stimulate an inflammatory/hypercoagulable state with platelet activation and remodeling of the vascular endothelium. The resulting clinical presentation is thrombocytopenia and a high risk of thrombosis in any venous or arterial site. This article summarizes the current knowledge in this area.

ANTIPHOSPHOLIPID SYNDROME

Among the identified acquired blood protein defects that are known to lead to thrombosis, APS is among the most common [3–8]. APS can be seen in association with systemic lupus erythematosus (SLE), connective tissue and autoimmune disorders, malignancy, HIV infection, and drug reactions. A common misconception is that patients who have drug-induced APS, often immunoglobulin (Ig) M, do not suffer thrombosis, but in fact they have an increased risk of thrombosis. Thrombotic events are reported in approximately 30% of patients who have APS, with an overall incidence of 2.5% patients/year (higher if there has been a past thrombotic episode).

*Corresponding author. E-mail address: jwaleng@lumc.edu (J.M. Walenga).

0889-8588/08/$ – see front matter © 2008 Elsevier Inc. All rights reserved.
doi:10.1016/j.hoc.2007.11.001 hemonc.theclinics.com

The great majority of individuals developing APS are otherwise healthy and harbor no other underlying medical conditions. The antibodies may be transient and asymptomatic. These otherwise healthy individuals are classified as having primary rather than secondary APS.

The family of antiphospholipid immunoglobulins is heterogeneous and targets a variety of potential antigenic targets. APS can be caused by the lupus anticoagulant (LA), anticardiolipin antibodies (ACA), or other antiphospholipid antibodies. ACA-associated thrombosis is more common than the LA-associated thrombosis, with a ratio of 5:1 [5]. Phospholipids are involved in many important processes throughout the hemostatic system. APS antibodies are associated with fetal wastage, arterial or venous thrombosis, and thrombocytopenia. There are distinct clinical, laboratory, and biochemical differences between the disorders mediated by the different antibodies.

Antiphospholipid Syndrome Antibodies

The antibodies that manifest as the APS can target phospholipids directly [5]. These anti-phospholipid antibodies (APAs) target cardiolipin, phosphatidylserine, phosphatidylinositol, phosphatidylethanolamine, phosphatidylglycerol, and phosphatidylcholine. APAs can be IgG, IgA, and IgM idiotypes. APAs are subgrouped based on type of antibody. The presence of APAs may be associated with either venous or arterial thrombosis [3–8].

APS can also be caused by antibodies that target protein antigens which bind to anionic phospholipids, forming a protein-phospholipid complex. The predominant antibodies in APS are those that target the proteins beta-2-glycoprotein I (β2-GPI) and prothrombin [9,10], although other antigenic targets have been identified in APS patients [11–15]. For example, antibodies against annexin V and protein C have been shown to be associated with APS and SLE.

The term LA is based on a laboratory artifact. Because this antibody interferes with the action of phospholipid cofactors in the coagulation cascade in laboratory assays, a prolongation of the time to clot is produced, mimicking an apparent anticoagulant response. This is a misnomer, because the presence of an LA is associated with clinical thrombosis and not bleeding [16,17]. Specifically, the LA inhibits the formation of the prothrombinase complex within the coagulation cascade. It blocks the binding of prothrombin and factor Xa to phospholipids, which inhibits the conversion of prothrombin to thrombin and clot formation [18]. The LA can be an IgG, IgA, or IgM. The LA is found in at least 10% of patients who have SLE and in many patients who have autoimmune disorders. LA is commonly associated with venous thrombosis and only occasionally with arterial disease.

Mechanism of Thrombosis in Antiphospholipid Syndrome

The precise mechanism whereby hemostasis is altered to induce a hypercoagulable state in APS remains unclear. Because the antibodies in APS are heterogeneous and more than one type is probably present in any given patient [5], several mechanisms may be responsible for the clinical manifestations in patients who have APS.

Because phospholipids are an integral part of platelet and endothelial cell surface membranes, it is expected that anti-phospholipid antibodies would have a significant effect on platelet and vascular endothelial mechanisms. The currently proposed mechanisms of action involve platelet activation, blood coagulation alterations, fibrinolytic deficit, endothelial cell remodeling, or combined effects. These mechanisms are described below.

Platelet activation

Antibodies to beta-2-glycoprotein I. β2-GPI is an inhibitor of contact activation of the coagulation system, the factor Xa-generating activity of platelets, and adenosine diphosphate (ADP)-induced platelet aggregation [19,20]. Following platelet activation, phospholipid binding proteins such as β2-GPI interact with the negatively charged phospholipids that are exposed on the surface of the platelet. The protein bound to phospholipid exposes normally cryptic epitopes on the phospholipid. These neoepitopes can induce antibody formation [9,10]. If antibodies to β2-GPI are formed, the natural anticoagulant properties of β2-GPI are blocked. Complexes of β2-GPI-phospholipid antibody activate platelets via binding to the FcγIIa platelet receptor, causing platelet activation and aggregation. Platelet activation leads to up-regulation of surface phospholipids and receptors advancing, further β2-GPI-phospholipid complex formation, antibody generation, and additional platelet and cellular activation, establishing a positive feedback cycle and the eventual formation of platelet-rich thrombi.

Interaction of platelets with endothelial cells. Platelets that have bound APAs alter platelet-endothelial cell interactions [21–27]. A recent study indicates that although endothelial activation occurs, it is the platelet activation that is significantly more enhanced in APS patients who have thrombosis compared with those who do not have thrombosis [26].

Another study demonstrated that both antigen and activity levels of von Willebrand factor (vWF; released from endothelial cells) are positively associated with thrombosis in APS patients [27]. The study authors suggest that vWF mediates increased platelet adhesion, and that this would complement the known ability of APS antibodies to enhance platelet response to agonists in conventional aggregometry.

Interaction of platelets with leukocytes. Activated platelets interact with leukocytes. In the presence of APAs, increased tissue factor (TF) expression from monocytes [28–30].

Anti-annexin V antibodies. Annexin V is a calcium-dependent vascular anticoagulant protein that binds to phospholipids, preferably phosphatidylserine (PS), on platelet membrane surfaces. Exposure of PS on the cell surfaces produces proinflammatory and procoagulant activities. Annexin V binds to PS, thus inhibiting these responses. Anti-annexin V antibodies interfere with the annexin V-induced inhibition of the procoagulant and proinflammatory activities of apoptotic cells [12]. High levels of anti-annexin V have been detected in patients who have SLE and APS, and have been associated with an increased risk of thrombosis that leads to recurrent abortions, pre-eclampsia, and fetal death [31–33].

Down-regulation of prostacyclin. Prostacyclin is an important inhibitor of platelet activation formed from arachidonic acid that is released from platelet and endothelial cell membrane phospholipids. There is evidence that APAs impair prostacyclin synthesis in endothelial cells and up-regulate the generation of thromboxane, leading to vasoconstriction and platelet aggregation [34–36].

Blood coagulation alterations
Reduced activity of protein C and protein S. Both protein C and protein S are important inhibitors of the coagulation system. Protein C and its cofactor protein S are bound to the thrombin-thrombomodulin complex that is bound to a negatively charged phospholipid surface. Because APAs interfere with the binding of the proteins to thrombomodulin, activation of protein C could be inhibited, or the activity of protein C could be inhibited [37]. Vascular damage may lead to the release of thrombomodulin, thus interfering in the regulatory functions mediated by the thrombin-thrombomodulin complex.

Interference with antithrombin III activity. Heparan sulfate on the surface of endothelial cells acts as a natural anticoagulant through binding with antithrombin III (AT). IgG isolated from patients who have APS reacts with a specific disaccharide sequence found in the critical AT binding region of heparin, heparan sulfate, and other glycosaminoglycans (GAGs) [38]. This may reduce the endogenous anticoagulant activity of AT, and it may also inhibit the release of tissue factor pathway inhibitor (TFPI) from endothelial cells. TFPI is a natural inhibitor of TF. The inhibition of TFPI release may be related to a conformational change of endothelial cells caused by an altered binding of GAGs.

Up-regulation of tissue factor expression. IgGs from patients who have LA induce TF activation in endothelial cell culture [39–41]. The expression of TF on endothelial cells induced by isolated IgG from LA patients has been shown to correlate with clinical thrombosis.

Fibrinolytic deficit. Binding of APAs to endothelial cells down-regulates the expression of tissue plasminogen activator (tPA), leading to a decrease in fibrinolytic activity [23,25,42]. An up-regulation of the inhibitor to tPA, plasminogen activator inhibitor (PAI-1), has also been shown in patients who have APA. Other fibrinolytic inhibitors such as thrombin activatable fibrinolytic inhibitor (TAFI) may be involved but have not yet been investigated.

Interference with endothelial cell phospholipids
Endothelial cells are involved in many of the hemostatic mechanisms, either directly or in combination with activated platelets, proteins, receptors, enzymes, and so forth. Potential mechanisms of hemostatic abnormalities associated with endothelial cells in APS (as described above) may be caused by prothrombotic endothelial cells. If β2-GPI binds to phospholipid on the vascular endothelial surface, circulating APAs will recognize and bind to the β2-GPI-phospholipid complex and cause endothelial cell damage. This can result in the exposure of endothelial substances of procoagulant activity such as TF.

Platelet-endothelial cell interactions and platelet-leukocyte interactions can be enhanced, augmenting the procoagulant state and establishing a site for thrombus formation. The natural anticoagulant substances expressed on the surface of normal endothelial cells are reduced because of the cellular injury, leading to blood coagulation activation with loss of fibrinolytic activity. Cytokines from the injured endothelium and activated leukocytes produce an inflammatory response that further damages the endothelium and promotes the procoagulant state.

Up-regulation of inflammation
Inflammation plays a major role in the pathogenesis of autoimmune diseases. Anti-annexin V antibodies are associated with inflammation and a procoagulant state [43]. Inflammation is intimately associated with the activation of the hemostatic system through endothelial cell interactions with cytokines that increase C-reactive protein (CRP), nitric oxide (NO), and other substances that subsequently up- or down-regulate the hemostatic factors. For example, tumor necrosis factor α (TNFα) induces TF expression from endothelial cells [40]. It has been shown that endothelial cells are activated by APAs, as demonstrated by an up-regulation of the adhesion molecules vascular cell adhesion molecule (VCAM) and E-selectin [22].

HEPARIN-INDUCED THROMBOCYTOPENIA
HIT is one of the most important life and limb-threatening adverse drug events [44,45]. It is described as an immune disorder associated with exposure to heparin. It occurs in approximately 2% of all patients exposed to heparin (frequency differs by patient population), of which approximately 35% develop thrombosis.

The frequency of developing HIT antibodies can be very high (eg, up to 40% in post-cardiac surgery patients [46–49]); however, the presence of HIT antibody alone does not necessarily correlate with clinical symptoms. Antibodies that are not associated with clinical symptoms have been termed "non-functional"; however, it may be that these are functional antibodies, but that all conditions have not been met to develop clinical symptoms. HIT antibodies typically remain in circulation for 90 days.

In the classical sense, HIT presents clinically with a marked thrombocytopenia, but can be mild and less apparent. Thrombocytopenia is temporally related to HIT antibody titer increase [50]. Platelet aggregation occurs when large numbers of platelets are activated. This results in a decreased number of free circulating platelets in the blood and increases the likelihood of platelet-rich clot formation. HIT may develop into arterial or venous thrombosis if heparin is not discontinued and the patient treated with alternate anticoagulation. Amputation may be necessary, and in severe cases death may ensue.

Heparin-Induced Thrombocytopenia Antibodies
The mechanism of HIT is based on antibody formation with the antigenic target of a complex of heparin bound to a specific protein, not to heparin alone.

Most often the protein in the complex is platelet factor 4 (PF4), a substance stored in platelet alpha granules [51–53]. Interleukin-8 (IL-8) and neutrophil-activating peptide-2 (NAP-2) have also been identified as protein antigens [54]. The PF4-heparin complex presents a neo-epitope on PF4, to which antibodies are generated. These can be IgG, IgM, or IgA antibodies.

The importance of PF4 as the immunogen for inducing HIT is becoming more clear with recent findings [55,56]. This is of interest when evaluating clinical outcomes. For example, so-called "delayed" HIT, or thrombocytopenia that occurs 10 or more days after heparin exposure (when the patient is at home as opposed to in the acute hospital setting), may be induced when the PF4 concentration increases because of pathologic activity related to cardiovascular, inflammatory, or another activation process. This also may explain why different patient populations are more prone to HIT and thrombosis than others.

The IgG antibodies determined by diagnostic laboratory assays such as the serotonin release assay (SRA) have been correlated with acute clinical symptoms, which is not unexpected if one considers the mechanism of the SRA [45,57,58]. The authors believe, however, that IgM and IgA antibodies are also important in HIT. IgM may be a marker of the initial phase of HIT. The development of IgG and thrombocytopenia are events that occur in a later phase of HIT, which, depending on the patient's overall status, may be too late to successfully manage. Thus once a patient converts to IgG, the clinical symptoms become much more evident, and therefore more serious. Moreover, it has been demonstrated that certain patients who have HIT clinical symptoms have only IgM or IgA antibodies without IgG antibodies (to the PF4-heparin complex) [53].

Mechanism of Thrombosis in Heparin-Induced Thrombocytopenia

HIT antibodies bind to PF4-heparin complexes and to FcγIIa receptors on platelets and endothelium. This causes platelet activation, platelet aggregation, and the formation of procoagulant platelet microparticles [59,60]. Platelet activation results in the release of more PF4 from platelet granules and a continuation of the platelet activation cycle. It can also be considered that glycosaminoglycans (GAGs; heparin, heparan sulfate) and PF4 are bound to the surface of platelets, and that these are up-regulated with platelet activation. This would enhance the platelet activation response.

HIT antibodies are involved in other hemostatic activation processes. Platelets activated by HIT antibodies induce an inflammatory state in which macrophages, monocytes, and neutrophils are activated [61]. Activated leukocytes bind to and interact with platelets via up-regulated platelet P-selectin [59,62,63]. TF and cytokines are released from activated monocytes and endothelial cells, and neutrophils show an increase in their metabolic activity and alterations in their cell surface adhesive receptors.

Microvascular and macrovascular endothelium have natural surface GAGs (mostly heparan sulfate). PF4 can bind to these GAGs, to which the HIT antibodies bind, causing local damage to the endothelium. Microvascular and macrovascular endothelial cell remodeling occurs in the presence of HIT antibodies and activated platelets [61]. Antibody and leukocyte binding to activated endothelial cells causes release of tissue factor, PAI-1, cytokines, and adhesion molecules from the endothelial cells [64–67]. This promotes localized platelet and monocyte binding to the vascular endothelium. Heparan sulfate on the endothelial cell surface can bind PF4 forming a complex that is recognized by HIT antibodies [68,69].

Vascular endothelial cells are adversely affected by HIT antibodies. Macrovascular endothelial cells (human umbilical vein endothelial cells [HUVEC])-incubated with heparin and serum from HIT patients results in a platelet dependent and time-dependent increase in the expression of PAI-1 and TF [64]. On the other hand, microvascular endothelial cells could be activated by isolated HIT immunoglobulin with no need for platelets or other stimuli [67]. These findings illustrate a differential effect in the ability of HIT antibodies to bind macrovascular and microvascular endothelial cells.

This combined cellular activation in HIT leads to a burst of thrombin generation with induction of a strong hypercoagulable state and inflammation [70]. The inter-relationships of platelets, leukocytes, the endothelium, and the inflammatory state determine the clinical expression of HIT.

COMMONALITIES BETWEEN ANTIPHOSPHOLIPID SYNDROME AND HEPARIN-INDUCED THROMBOCYTOPENIA
Clinical Presentations
In both APS and HIT, the clinical presentation is similar. Many patients can harbor antibody without having clinical signs or symptoms of the disorder. When a reaction does occur, the clinical presentation of APS and HIT is similar in terms of thrombocytopenia and high risk of thrombosis. In both cases catastrophic clinical outcomes have been commonly reported, particularly if the disorder was not treated early [44,71]. APS often presents as a chronic and mild condition; HIT can have a mild presentation too, although it is more often an acute reaction.

In APS and HIT the threshold for thrombogenesis is lowered. Patients who have APS are reported to have premature coronary occlusion, cerebrovascular disease, hepatic vein, portal vein, mesenteric artery, renal vein, retinal vein, and upper limb thrombosis, stroke, myocardial infarction, aorto-coronary graft closure, and reocclusion of post-angioplasty vessels [5–7,17,28,29,31–33,72,73]. Renal artery, mesenteric arteries, upper limb, cardiac, and cerebral sinus thrombosis have been identified in HIT patients [44]. Deep venous thrombosis and pulmonary embolism are the most frequent clinical syndromes identified in patients who have either APS or HIT [3,5–7,44]. In both disorders vessels in any organ and any size vessel can be affected.

The one exception is that APS patients often experience recurrent fetal loss that is not observed in HIT patients.

In both APS and HIT, IgG is most often associated with thrombosis; however, there are cases of patients who have only IgM antibodies who experience thrombosis. In APS the IgM-mediated thrombosis is most often related to drug ingestion.

The site of thrombosis seems to depend on patient-related factors in both APS and HIT. In addition, in both disorders, when antibodies are present the association with other risk factors may cause a thrombotic event. Both APS and HIT can be associated with the "double hit" theory applied to thrombosis risk. Both disorders often occur in the presence of an underlying disease such as malignancy, or with an infection, inflammation, or trauma.

To avoid serious complications, it is advised to commence anticoagulation treatment of patients who have APS or HIT upon initial clinical suspicion of the disorder. Treatment is obviously different for the two disorders because heparin and low molecular weight heparin (LMWH) cannot be given to patients who have HIT, and alternative anticoagulation with a direct thrombin inhibitor is the current treatment of choice [45]. On the other hand, LMWH is the current treatment of choice for APS [5].

Pathological Mechanism

As the mechanism of action of APS and HIT becomes better understood, it appears that both disorders share a commonality in their pathogenic mechanism. This has been suggested in previous publications [1,2,65]. In both HIT and APS antibodies target vascular sites and platelets. These antibodies induce inflammation, a hypercoagulable state, thrombocytopenia, and thrombosis (Box 1). In both disorders there remains debate whether the target of cellular injury is predominately platelets or endothelial cells.

Immune-mediated response

Both the APS and HIT syndromes are autoimmune disorders. The causative antibodies of APS and HIT are distinct; however, in both disorders the antibody targets a bound protein. Normally cryptic epitopes on the protein (β2-GPI for APS and PF4 for HIT) are exposed after it binds to a natural substrate (phospholipid or heparin/heparan, respectively). These neoepitopes induce antibody formation; the antigen-antibody complex binds to and activates FcγIIa receptors, resulting in platelet activation and perturbations of vascular endothelial cells.

These patients are in an exaggerated state of immune response. It is hypothesized that patients who have APS can simultaneously develop HIT and that HIT patients can simultaneously develop APS. In fact, it has been shown that APAs from patients who have APS bind to heparin [14], and autoantibodies to heparan sulfate have been identified at the site of vascular injury in patients who have SLE and renal disease [38].

Platelet activation occurs in patients who have APS, and with it PF4 is released. This PF4 can bind to heparan sulfate on endothelial cells, and this complex could trigger the generation of HIT antibodies (Fig. 1). This process could be augmented if the APS patient is treated with heparin (unfractionated heparin would be a stronger stimulant than LMWH). Conversely, it is

> **Box 1: Similar pathophysiologic mechanisms in APS and HIT**
>
> *Autoimmune response*
>
> *Generation of antibodies to a bound protein antigen complex*
>
> *Hemostatic activation processes associated with antibody production*
> Procoagulant state
>   TF release
>   Thrombin generation
> Platelet activation
>   Procoagulant platelet microparticle formation
>   Platelet release reaction
>   Platelet adhesion
>   Platelet aggregation
> Leukocyte activation
>   Monocytes and neutrophils bind to platelets
>   Leukocytes release TF, cytokines, and so forth
> Remodeling of endothelial cells
>   Antibodies bind to cells
>   Cells are altered to a procoagulant state
>   Site for thrombus is established
>
> *Pro-inflammatory state*
> Up-regulation of cytokines
> Up-regulation of inflammatory mediators
> Up-regulation of adhesion molecules

hypothesized that a simultaneous generation of APAs could develop in patients who have HIT (Fig. 2). HIT antibodies cause vascular damage that could result in configurational changes in membrane phospholipids of the endothelial cells. These alterations could lead to the generation of APAs.

In a study by the authors and colleagues, it has been shown that anti-annexin V antibodies are consistently elevated in both APS and HIT patients [74]. Several authors have shown positive testing of both PF4-heparin antibodies and APAs in patients [75–77]. Whether the double antibody represents an additional risk factor for the development of thrombotic complications in these patient populations or whether there is a cross-reaction between tests causing false-positive results is unknown. There may be an interaction between APAs, HIT antibodies, and their disease processes.

In addition, it is known that HIT antibodies can be targeted to inflammatory proteins (IL-8, NAP-2) [54]. It should be investigated in patients who have APS whether these same types of antibodies exist in this disorder as well. Because of

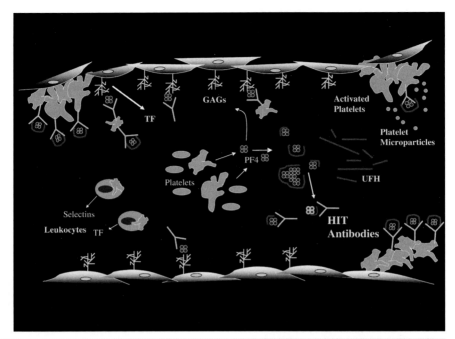

Fig. 1. Proposed mechanism of the generation of PF4-heparin antibodies in patients who have APS. In APS patients, distorted vascular endothelium leads to the exposure of GAGs such as heparan sulfate that may complex with PF4, which is generated from activated platelets. Heparan sulfate complexes with PF4, causing allosteric modifications in the PF4 molecule, transforming it into a neo-antigen. This can lead to the generation of PF4-heparin antibodies.

the heightened inflammatory state in APS and HIT patients, it is possible that there are related antibodies in these two disorders associated with inflammation.

Biomarkers of hemostatic activation
The similarity between APS and HIT is supported by studies that demonstrate similar findings between the two patient populations in terms of biological indicators of a hypercoagulable and inflammatory state. The authors and others have evaluated biomarkers related to the pathogenesis of thrombosis, including thrombin generation, fibrinolysis, platelet activation, endothelial cell function, and inflammation in patients who have either APS or HIT. Diagnosis was determined by clinical symptoms and specific antibody assays. The findings are summarized below (Box 2).

Biomarkers of thrombin generation. In APS and HIT patients, thrombin generation is significantly enhanced [65].

Biomarkers of platelet activation. Soluble P-selectin levels and complexes of platelets with leukocytes were significantly elevated in both HIT and APS patients, indicating significant platelet activation in both disease states [65].

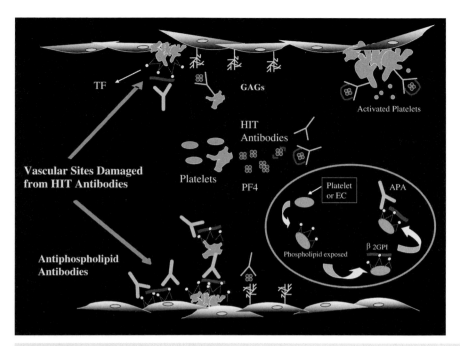

Fig. 2. Proposed mechanism of the generation of APAs in patients who have HIT. The formation of APAs in HIT patients may be secondary to the vascular damage produced by HIT antibodies, which exposes endothelial cell membrane phospholipids, thereby triggering the formation of APAs. Vascular damage and configurational changes in endothelial cell membranes result in phospholipids that induce the generation of APAs in APS. The composition of phospholipids determines the type of antibodies.

Biomarkers of endothelial dysfunction. Elevated levels of soluble thrombomodulin (s-TM) and TF were observed, indicating that the vascular endothelium is disrupted or damaged in both HIT and APS patients [65,74]. s-TM levels were higher in HIT than APS patients, whereas TF levels were higher in APS than HIT patients studied. In both groups, TF levels were higher in patients who had thrombosis compared with those who did not have thrombosis. The variable levels of the biomarkers may relate to different degrees of pathogenesis rather than a difference between APS and HIT. Levels of vWF did not differ between groups or from normal.

Biomarkers of inflammation. There was a significant increase in the level of CRP in both HIT and APS patients, demonstrating a role of inflammation in the pathogenesis of HIT and APS. TNFα was elevated in many of the APS and HIT patients. All of the HIT patients and most of the APS patients had elevated IL-6 levels [65,74].

CD40L is a member of the TNF cytokine family that binds to endothelial cells, monocytes, and other cells affecting isotype switching, cytokine

> **Box 2: Biomarkers of antibody-mediated hemostatic activation in both APS and HIT**
>
> Hypercoagulable state
>   Thrombin generation
>   AT
>   Heparin cofactor II (HC II)
>   protein C
>   protein S
>   TF
>   TFPI
>   TAFI
>   PAI-1
>
> Platelet activation
>   Platelet microparticles
>   Soluble P-selectin
>   Platelet-leukocyte binding
>
> Endothelial dysfunction related to procoagulant activity
>   vWF
>   PAI-1
>   TF
>   Soluble thrombomodulin (s-TM)
>
> Inflammation
>   Cytokines
>   NO
>   CRP
>   CD-40 ligand (CD40L)
>   Leukocyte activation

production, amplification of the inflammatory state, and thrombin activation of platelets [78]. Soluble CD40L is up-regulated in most APS and HIT patients [65,79,80].

SUMMARY

APS and HIT are two autoimmune disorders caused by distinct antibodies; however, as studied to date, the immune mechanism shares a certain degree of similarity (Boxes 3 and 4). In both disorders the target antigen is a bound protein (to either phospholipid in APS or to heparin in HIT).

> **Box 3: Clinical commonalities between APS and HIT**
>
> Patients can harbor antibody without any clinical symptom
>
> There is commonly an underlying disorder that stimulates the autoimmune response (infection, trauma, malignancy)
>
> Patients have a similar inflammatory response (see Boxes 1 and 2)
>
> Patients have a similar hypercoagulable state/thrombin generation (see Boxes 1 and 2)
>
> Similar antibodies may be generated in each (simultaneous HIT antibodies and APAs)
>
> Patients are at high risk of morbidity and mortality
>
> Thrombosis can occur in any size vessel, of any organ, in any vascular bed
>
> Severe and catastrophic thrombotic complications can occur
>
> Deep vein thrombosis and pulmonary embolism are the most common thrombotic complications
>
> Patients require anticoagulation
>
>   Treatment should be initiated when disorder is suspected
>
>   Aspirin is not very effective
>
>   Warfarin failures are common

It should also be considered that because of the pathology that the antibodies induce on the vascular endothelium, there could be simultaneous generation of APAs in patients who have HIT and generation of HIT antibodies in patients who have APS. There is suggestive evidence that anti-annexin V antibodies occur in both APS and HIT, and also evidence of patients who have combined APAs and HIT antibodies. PF4 from platelet activation occurs in both APS and

> **Box 4: Clinical differences between APS and HIT**
>
> In addition to the β2-GPI antibodies, there is a heterogeneous mixture of other antibody types that cause APS (antibodies that bind directly to various phospholipids; the lupus anticoagulant)
>
> There are clinical, biochemical, and diagnostic laboratory differences for each of the different APS antibody-mediated diseases
>
> Fetal wastage only occurs with APS
>
> Central nervous system-related symptoms (behavior disturbances, grand mal seizures) and other broad-based, diverse symptoms only occur with APS
>
> Anticoagulation treatments differ
>
>   APS: treatment with low molecular weight heparin and the antiplatelet drug clopidogrel
>
>   HIT: treatment with a non-heparin anticoagulant (direct thrombin inhibitors)

HIT. Alteration of platelet and endothelial bound phospholipids could occur in both APS and HIT via damage from the antibodies. Thus the one disorder may enhance the physiological setting for stimulation of the other.

A combined inflammatory/procoagulant state exists in both APS and HIT patients. There is direct activation of platelets and endothelial cells by the antibodies in both APS and HIT. In addition a similar inflammatory response exists in APS and HIT. The pathological inflammatory response is likely the primary event that occurs before more complex hemostatic system alterations are induced. The pathogenesis of hemostatic activation in both disorders centers on cellular dysfunction, with subsequent aberrations to the hemostatic network.

Perhaps the most important aspect of the common pathophysiology of APS and HIT is the vascular pathogenesis that these disorders share. A costimulatory situation exists in both disorders, which is increased vascular damage caused by excess immune complex formation, leading to strong thrombin generation and thrombosis. Evidence of platelet activation, fibrinolytic deficit, and thrombin generation has been described in both APS and HIT patients. Substances such as cytokines generated from the inflammatory process can serve as a link between inflammation and hypercoagulability, promoting platelet-mediated endothelial cell activation, platelet-leukocyte interactions, and production of procoagulant substances from endothelial cells and platelets, and the like.

For both APS and HIT there is often a poor correlation between clinical laboratory tests and clinical findings. This may be because there are many different laboratory tests, and some tests are more sensitive than others. Perhaps the true pathophysiology and chosen laboratory markers being used for diagnostic testing are not optimal. As the pathophysiological mechanisms of APS and HIT are better understood, improved diagnostic measures may be developed that can be used to identify individual patients at higher risk of morbidity or mortality, or as indicators to guide therapeutic intervention. In addition, recent findings suggest that in addition to anticoagulation treatment, both APS and HIT patients may benefit from anti-inflammatory and anti-platelet adjunctive therapy.

References

[1] Arnout J. The pathogenesis of the antiphospholipid syndrome: a hypothesis based on parallelisms with heparin-induced-thrombocytopenia. Thromb Haemost 1996;75(4): 536–41.
[2] Vermylen J, Hoylaerts JF, Arnout J. Antibody-mediated thrombosis. Thromb Haemost 1997;78(1):420–6.
[3] Bick RL, Jakway J, Baker WF. Deep vein thrombosis: prevalence of etiologic factors and results of management in 100 consecutive patients. Semin Thromb Hemost 1992;18: 267–74.
[4] Bick RL, Baker WF. Anticardiolipin antibodies and thrombosis. Hematol Oncol Clin North Am 1992;6:1287–99.
[5] Bick RL. Antiphospholipid thrombosis syndromes. Hematol Oncol Clin North Am 2003;17(1):115–47.

[6] Kunkel LA. Acquired circulating anticoagulants. Hematol Oncol Clin North Am 1992;6: 1341–57.
[7] Alving BM. Antiphospholipid syndrome, lupus anticoagulants, and anticardiolipin antibodies. In: Loscalzo J, Schafer AI, editors. Thrombosis and hemorrhage. 2nd edition. Baltimore: Williams & Wilkins; 1998. p. 817–33.
[8] Triplett DA. Antiphospholipid antibodies and thrombosis. A consequence, coincidence, or cause? Arch Pathol Lab Med 1993;117:78–88.
[9] Bevers EM, Galli M, Barbui T, et al. Lupus anticoagulant IgG's are not directed to phospholipids only, but to a complex of lipid-bound human prothrombin. Thromb Haemost 1991;66: 629–32.
[10] McNeil HP, Simpson RJ, Chesterman CN. Anti-phospholipid antibodies are directed against a complex antigen that includes a lipid-binding inhibitor of coagulation: β2-glycoprotein I (apolipoprotein H). Proc Natl Acad Sci U S A 1990;87:4120–4.
[11] Matsuura E, Igarashi Y, Fujimoto M, et al. Anticardiolipin cofactor(s) and differential diagnosis of autoimmune disease. Lancet 1990;336:177–8.
[12] Nakamura N, Kuragaki C, Shidara Y, et al. Antibody to annexin V has anti-phospholipid and lupus anticoagulant properties. Am J Hematol 1995;49:347–8.
[13] Oosting JD, Derksen RHWM, Bobbick IWG, et al. Antiphospholipid antibodies directed against a combination of phospholipids with prothrombin, protein C or protein S. An explanation for their pathogenic mechanism. Blood 1993;81:2618–25.
[14] Shibata S, Harpel PC, Gharavi A, et al. Autoantibodies to heparin from patients with antiphospholipid antibody syndrome inhibits formation of antithrombin III-thrombin complexes. Blood 1994;83:2532–40.
[15] Galli M. Non beta 2-glycoprotein I cofactors for antiphospholipid antibodies. Lupus 1996;5:388–92.
[16] Bowie EJW, Thompson JH, Pascuzzi CA, et al. Thrombosis in systemic lupus erythematosus despite circulating anticoagulants. J Lab Clin Med 1963;62:416–30.
[17] Alarcon-Segovia D. Clinical manifestations of the antiphospholipid syndrome. J Rheumatol 1992;18:1916–8.
[18] Triplett DA. Protean clinical presentation of antiphospholipid-protein antibodies (APA). Thromb Haemost 1995;74(1):329.
[19] She W, Chong BH, Hogg PJ, et al. Anticardiolipin antibodies block the inhibition of 2 GPI of the factor Xa generating activity of platelets. Thromb Haemost 1993;70:342–5.
[20] Nimpf J, Wurm H, Kostner GM. Beta 2 glycoprotein I (apo-H) inhibits the release reaction of human platelets during ADP-induced aggregation. Atherosclerosis 1987;63:109–14.
[21] Maruyama I. Biology of endothelium. Lupus 1998;7:S41–3.
[22] Pierangeli SS, Coleen-Stanfield M, Liu X, et al. Antiphospholipid antibodies from antiphospholipid syndrome patients' active endothelial cells in vitro and in vivo. Circulation 1999;99:1997–2002.
[23] LeRoux G, Wautier MP, Guillevin L, et al. IgG binding to endothelial cells in systemic lupus erythematosus. Thromb Haemost 1986;56:144–6.
[24] Hasselaar P, Derksen RHWM, Blokzijl L, et al. Cross reactivity of antibodies directed against cardiolipin, DNA, endothelial cells and blood platelets. Thromb Haemost 1990;63:169–73.
[25] Angles-Cano E, Sultan Y, Clauvel JP. Predisposing factors to thrombosis in systemic lupus erythematosus: possible relation to endothelial damage. J Lab Clin Med 1979;94: 317–23.
[26] Bidot CJ, JY W, Horstman LL, et al. Antiphospholipid antibodies and platelet activation as risk factors for thrombosis in thrombocythaemia. Hematology 2005;10(6):451–6.
[27] Levy Y, Shenkman B, Tamarin I, et al. Increased platelet deposition on extracellular matrix under flow conditions in patients with antiphospholipid syndrome who experience thrombotic events. Arthritis Rheum 2005;52(12):4011–7.
[28] Gavaghan TP, Krilis SA, Daggard GE. Anticardiolipin antibodies and occlusion of coronary artery bypass grafts. Lancet 1987;2(8565):977–8.

[29] Baker WF, Bick RL. Antiphospholipid antibodies in coronary artery disease: a review. Semin Thromb Hemost 1994;20(1):27–45.
[30] Reverter JC, Tassies D, Font J, et al. Hypercoagulable state in patients with antiphospholipid syndrome is related to high induced tissue factor expression on monocytes and to low free protein S. Arterioscler Thromb Vasc Biol 1996;16:1319–26.
[31] Kaburaki J, Kuwana M, Yamamoto M, et al. Clinical significance of anti-annexin V antibodies in patients with systemic lupus erythematosus. Am J Hematol 1997;54:209–13.
[32] Nakamura N, Shidara Y, Kawaguchi N, et al. Lupus anticoagulant autoantibody induces apoptosis in umbilical vein endothelial cells: involvement of annexin V. Biochem Biophys Res Commun 1994;205:1488–93.
[33] Matsuda J, Gotoh M, Saith M, et al. Anti-annexin antibody in the sera of patients with habitual fetal loss or preeclampsia. Thromb Res 1994;75:105–6.
[34] Carreras LO, Defreyn G, Machin SJ, et al. Arterial thrombosis, intrauterine death and "lupus" anticoagulant: detection of immunoglobulin interfering with prostacyclin formation. Lancet 1981;I(8214):244–6.
[35] Martinuzzo ME, Maclouf J, Carreras LO, et al. Antiphospholipid antibodies enhance thrombin induced platelet activation and thromboxane formation. Thromb Haemost 1993;70:667–71.
[36] Rustin MHA, Bull HA, Machin SJ, et al. Effects of lupus anticoagulant in patients with systemic lupus erythematosus on endothelial cells prostacyclin release and procoagulant activity. J Invest Dermatol 1988;90:744–8.
[37] Smirov MD, Triplett DA, Comp PC, et al. On the role of phosphatidylethanolamine in the inhibition of activated protein C activity by antiphospholipid antibodies. J Clin Invest 1995;95:309–16.
[38] Pengo V, Biasiolo A, Grazia-Fior M. Binding of autoimmune cardiolipin-reactive antibodies to heparin: a mechanism of thrombosis? Thromb Res 1995;78(5):371–8.
[39] Tannenbaum SH, Finko R, Cines DB. Antibody and immune complexes induce tissue factor production by human endothelial cells. J Immunol 1986;137:1532–7.
[40] Ryan J, Brett J, Tijburg P, et al. Tumor necrosis factor induced endothelial tissue factor is associated with subendothelial matrix vesicles but is not expressed on the apical surface. Blood 1992;80:966–79.
[41] Brandt JT. The effects of lupus anticoagulant on the expression of tissue factor activity by cultured endothelial cells. Thromb Haemost 1991;65:673.
[42] Leurs J, Wissing B, Nerme V, et al. Different mechanisms contribute to the biphasic pattern of carboxypeptidase U (TAFIa) generation during in vitro clot lysis in human plasma. Thromb Haemost 2003;89:264–71.
[43] Reutelingsperger CP, van Heerde WL. Annexin V, the regulator of phosphatidylserine-catalyzed inflammation and coagulation during apoptosis. Cell Mol Life Sci 1997;53:527–32.
[44] Warkentin TE, Greinacher A. Heparin-induced thrombocytopenia: recognition, treatment, and prevention. Chest 2004;126:311S–37S.
[45] Walenga JM. Heparin-induced thrombocytopenia and treatment with thrombin inhibitors. Japanese Journal of Thrombosis and Hemostasis 2005;16(6):623–40.
[46] Pouplard C, May MA, Iochmann S, et al. Antibodies to platelet factor 4 heparin after cardiopulmonary bypass in patients anticoagulated with unfractionated heparin or a low molecular weight heparin: clinical implications for HIT. Circulation 1999;99:2530–6.
[47] Lindhoff-Last E, Eichler P, Stein M, et al. A prospective study on the incidence and clinical relevance of heparin-induced antibodies in patients after vascular surgery. Thromb Res 2000;97:387–93.
[48] Bauer TL, Arepally G, Konkle BA, et al. Prevalence of heparin-associated antibodies without thrombosis in patients undergoing cardiopulmonary bypass surgery. Circulation 1997;95:1242–6.

[49] Gluckman TJ, Segal JB, Fredde NL, et al. Incidence of anti-platelet factor 4/heparin antibody induction in patients undergoing percutaneous coronary revascularization. Am J Cardiol 2005;95:744–7.
[50] Kelton JG. The pathophysiology of heparin-induced thrombocytopenia. Chest 2005;127(2):9S–20S.
[51] Amiral J, Bridey F, Dreyfus M, et al. PF4 complexed to heparin is the target for antibodies generated in heparin-induced thrombocytopenia. Thromb Haemost 1992;68:95–6.
[52] Greinacher A, Pötzsch B, Amiral J, et al. Heparin-associated thrombocytopenia: isolation of the antibody and characterization of a multimolecular PF4-heparin complex as the major antigen. Thromb Haemost 1994;71:247–51.
[53] Amiral J, Wolf M, Fischer A-M, et al. Pathogenicity of IgA and/or IgM antibodies to heparin-PF4 complexes in patients with heparin-associated thrombocytopenia. Br J Haematol 1996;92:954.
[54] Amiral J, Marfaing-Koka A, Wolf M, et al. Presence of auto-antibodies to interleukin-8 or neutrophil activating peptide-2 in patients with heparin-associated thrombocytopenia. Blood 1996;88:410–6.
[55] Prechel MM, McDonald MK, Jeske WP, et al. Activation of platelets by heparin-induced thrombocytopenia antibodies in the serotonin release assay is not dependent on the presence of heparin. J Thromb Haemost 2005;3(10):2168–75.
[56] Prechel MM, Jeske WP, Walenga JM. Platelet-bound PF4 is targeted by HIT antibodies in the absence of heparin. Thromb Haemost 2007;5(Suppl 2):P-W-336.
[57] Ahmad S, Haas S, Hoppensteadt DA, et al. Differential effects of clivarin and heparin in patients undergoing hip and knee surgery for the generation of anti-heparin-platelet factor 4 antibodies. Thromb Res 2003;108:49–55.
[58] Prechel M, Jeske WP, Walenga JM. Laboratory methods for heparin-induced thrombocytopenia. In: Mousa SA, editor. Anticoagulants, antiplatelets, and thrombolytics: methods in molecular medicine. Totowa (NJ): Humana Press; 2004. p. 83–93.
[59] Jeske WP, Walenga JM, Szatkowski E, et al. Effect of glycoprotein IIb/IIIa antagonists on the HIT serum induced activation of platelets. Thromb Res 1997;88:271–81.
[60] Warkentin TE, Hayward CPM, Boshkov LK, et al. Sera from patients with heparin-induced thrombocytopenia generate platelet-derived microparticles with procoagulant activity: an explanation for the thrombotic complications of heparin-induced thrombocytopenia. Blood 1994;84:3691–9.
[61] Walenga JM, Jeske WP, Prechel MM, et al. Newer insights on the mechanism of heparin-induced thrombocytopenia. Semin Thromb Hemost 2004;30(Suppl 1):57–67.
[62] Jeske WP, Vasaiwala S, Schlenker R, et al. Leukocyte activation in heparin-induced thrombocytopenia. Blood 2000;96(11):29b.
[63] Pouplard C, Lochmann S, Renard B, et al. Induction of monocyte tissue factor expression by antibodies to heparin-platelet factor 4 complexes developed in heparin-induced thrombocytopenia. Blood 2001;97(10):3300–2.
[64] Herbert JM, Savi P, Jeske WP, et al. Effect of SR121566A, a potent GPIIb/IIIa antagonist, on the HIT serum/heparin-induced platelet mediated activation of human endothelial cells. Thromb Haemost 1998;80:326–31.
[65] Walenga JM, Michal K, Hoppensteadt D, et al. Vascular damage correlates between heparin-induced thrombocytopenia and the antiphospholipid syndrome. Clin Appl Thromb Hemost 1999;5(Suppl 1):S76–84.
[66] Fareed J, Walenga JM, Hoppensteadt DA, et al. Selectins in the HIT syndrome: pathophysiologic role and therapeutic modulation. Semin Thromb Hemost 1999;25(Suppl 1):37–42.
[67] Blank M, Shoenfeld Y, Tavor S, et al. Anti-platelet factor 4/heparin antibodies from patients with heparin-induced thrombocytopenia provoke direct activation of microvascular endothelial cells. Int Immunol 2002;14(2):121–9.

[68] Visentin GP, Ford SE, Scott PJ, et al. Antibodies from patients with heparin-induced thrombocytopenia/thrombosis are specific for platelet factor 4 complexed with heparin or bound to endothelial cells. J Clin Invest 1994;93:81–8.
[69] Suh JS, Aster RH, Visentin GP. Antibodies from patients with heparin-induced thrombocytopenia recognize different epitopes on heparin:platelet factor 4. Blood 1998;91:916–22.
[70] Walenga JM, Jeske WP, Messmore HL. Mechanisms of venous and arterial thrombosis in heparin-induced thrombocytopenia. J Thromb Thrombolysis 2000;10:S13–20.
[71] Shames DS, Broderick PA. Catastrophic antiphospholipid antibody syndrome. Conn Med 2001;65(1):3–5.
[72] Hess D. Stroke associated with antiphospholipid antibodies. Stroke 1992;23(Suppl 1): 123–8.
[73] Toschi V, Motta A, Castelli C, et al. High prevalence of antiphospholipid antibodies in young patients with cerebral ischemia of undetermined cause. Stroke 1998;29(9):1759–64.
[74] Baugh MJ, Prechel M, Hoppensteadt D, et al. The role of CD40 ligand and anti-annexin V antibodies in the pathophysiology of APS and HIT. Blood 2000;96(11):272a.
[75] Lasne D, Saffroy R, Bachelot C, et al. Tests for heparin-induced thrombocytopenia in primary antiphospholipid syndrome [abstract]. Br J Haematol 1997;97:939.
[76] de Larranaga G, Martinuzzo M, Bocassi A, et al. Heparin-platelet factor 4 induced antibodies in patients with either autoimmune or alloimmune antiphospholipid antibodies. Thromb Haemost 2002;88:371–3.
[77] Martin-Toutain I, Piette JC, Diemert MC. High prevalence of antibodies to platelet factor 4 heparin in patients with antiphospholipid antibodies in absence of heparin-induced thrombocytopenia. Lupus 2007;16:79–83.
[78] Van Kooten C, Banchereau J. CD40-CD40 ligand. J Leukoc Biol 2000;67:2–17.
[79] Desai-Mehta A, Lu L, Ramsey-Goldman R, et al. Hyperexpression of CD40 ligand by B and T cells in human lupus and its role in pathogenic autoantibody production. J Clin Invest 1996;97:2063–73.
[80] Koshy M, Berger D, Crow MK. Increased expression of CD40 Ligand on systemic lupus erythematosus lymphocytes. J Clin Invest 1996;98:826–37.

HEMATOLOGY/ONCOLOGY CLINICS OF NORTH AMERICA

Laboratory Evaluation of the Antiphospholipid Syndrome

Debra A. Hoppensteadt, PhD, SH, MT(ASCP)[a],*,
Nancy Fabbrini, MT(ASCP)[b], Rodger L. Bick, MD, PhD[c],
Harry L. Messmore, MD[d], Cafar Adiguzel, MD[d],
Jawed Fareed, PhD, FAHA[e,f]

[a]Department of Pathology, Stritch School of Medicine, Loyola University Chicago, 2160 S. First Avenue, Maywood, IL 60153, USA
[b]Department of Pathology, Edward Hines VA Hospital, Hines, IL, USA
[c]10455 North Central Expressway, Suite 109-320, Dallas, TX 75231, USA
[d]Department of Pathology, Loyola University Chicago, 2160 S. First Avenue, Maywood, IL 60153, USA
[e]Department of Pathology and Pharmacology, Loyola University Chicago, 2160 S. First Avenue, Maywood, IL 60153, USA
[f]Department of Cardiovascular Surgery, Loyola University Chicago, 2160 S. First Avenue, Maywood, IL 60153, USA

Patients recognized as being at increased risk for thrombosis have been referred to as having a "hypercoagulable state" or "thrombophilia." Box 1 lists the acquired blood protein defects that have been identified as leading to thrombosis [1]. Antiphospholipid syndrome (APLS) is among the most common acquired blood protein defects associated with thrombosis. APLS includes the lupus anticoagulant (LAC) and anticardiolipin antibodies (ACAs) and the recently recognized subgroups compromised of antibodies to β_2-glycoprotein I (β_2-GpI), phosphatidylserine, phosphatidylethanolamine, phosphatidylglycerol, phosphatidylinositol, phosphatidylcholine, and anti-annexin-V [1,2]. The presence of these antibodies, which may be associated with venous thrombosis, arterial thrombosis, or both, is more predictable than that observed in patients who have LAC [2].

Although ACAs and LAC have similarities, there are distinct clinical, laboratory, and biochemical differences, especially regarding prevalence, origin, possible mechanisms, clinical presentation, laboratory diagnosis, and management. The ACA syndrome is much more common than the LAC syndrome, the ratio being 5 or 6 to 1 [2]. Both syndromes may be associated with fetal wastage and thrombocytopenia. In addition, 5% to 15% of patients who have recurrent arterial and venous thrombosis have APLS [3]. In 50% of patients who have

*Corresponding author. E-mail address: dhoppen@lumc.edu (D.A. Hoppensteadt).

0889-8588/08/$ – see front matter © 2008 Elsevier Inc. All rights reserved.
doi:10.1016/j.hoc.2007.10.009   hemonc.theclinics.com

> **Box 1: The thrombophilias: hereditary and acquired blood coagulation protein and platelet defects**
>
> Antiphospholipid syndrome
>   Activated protein C resistance
>   Factor V Leiden
> Antithrombin deficiency
>   Protein C deficiency
>   Protein S deficiency
>   Factor V Cambridge
> Factor V Hong-Kong 1 & 2
>   Factor V HR2
>   Prothrombin G20210A
> Plasminogen activator inhibitor type 1 elevation/polymorphism
>   Methylene tetrahydrofolate reductase mutations
>   Homocysteinemia
>   Tissue plasminogen activator defects
> Heparin cofactor II defects
>   Factor XII defects
>   Dysfibrinogenemia
>   Immune vasculitis

systemic lupus, autoimmune antiphospholipid antibodies (APAs) have been detected [3,4]. Autoimmune antibodies also have been detected in rheumatoid arthritis and Sjögren's syndrome. Most individuals developing APLS are otherwise healthy and harbor no other underlying medical conditions [2–4].

APAs can develop in response to bacterial, viral, fungal, or parasitic infections and disappear within 12 weeks. These transient alloimmune antibodies have no clinical consequences [3], but they should be followed to determine persistence. The autoimmune APAs arise in collagen vascular diseases and can be associated with thrombosis.

Interest in antiphospholipids began in 1952 with the discovery of the LAC in about 10% of patients who had systemic lupus [5]. It was recognized that the presence of the LAC was associated with thrombosis instead of bleeding. It also was soon recognized that many patients who did not have autoimmune disorders harbored LAC. A common misconception is that patients who have drug-induced APLS (often IgM) do not suffer thrombosis; in fact they have an increased risk of developing thrombosis [2–4]. A number of other clinical reports confirmed the association of LAC and ACA with thromboembolic disease [6–8].

Because of a noted association of lupus, a biologic false-positive test for syphilis, and the presence of LAC, Harris and coworkers devised a new test for antiphospholipids using cardiolipin [9]. This and subsequent modifications now have become known as the "ACA test"; IgG, IgA and IgM anticardiolipin idiotypes are assessed. Shortly after the development of ACA assays, it became apparent that these antibodies are not limited to the population of patients who had LAC but are found in otherwise normal individuals as well [10,11]. The precise mechanisms whereby APAs alter hemostasis to induce a hypercoagulable state remain unclear, but several theories have been proposed. ACAs have affinity for phospholipids involved at many points in the hemostasis system. They are directed primarily against phosphatidylserine and phosphatidylinositol. Purified LAC, however, is capable of inhibiting the Ca^{2+} binding of prothrombin and coagulation factor Xa to phospholipids (prothrombinase complex), thereby inhibiting the activity of the phospholipid complex required for the conversion of prothrombin to thrombin [3]. The proposed mechanisms of action by which APLS interferes with hemostasis resulting in thrombosis are

- Reduced endothelial synthesis of prostacyclin
- Reduced activation of protein C via thrombomodulin/thrombin or interference with protein S activity, a cofactor to protein C activation
- Modulation of anticoagulant actions of antithrombin III activity
- Interaction with platelet membrane phospholipids leading to platelet activation and release
- Interference with activation of prekallikrein to kallikrein, which in turn activates the fibrinolytic system [12]
- Reduction of the release of endothelial cell plasminogen activator, thereby producing a fibrinolytic deficit and enhancing the key player of the fibrinolytic system

Endothelial cell–induced expression of tissue factor and antibodies to β_2-GpI also has been identified in patients who have APLS [1,2,10].

Extracellular annexin-V provides an antigenic stimulus for autoantibody formation [13]. The annexin-V is "flip-flopped" to the outer membrane surface where it is exposed to the APA [14]. It is thought that APAs form in response to newly formed complexes of protein and phospholipids [15,16]. High levels of anti-annexin-V have been detected in patients who have systemic lupus erythematosus and have been associated with an increase in thrombosis [14]. Anti-annexin-V autoantibodies from patients who have LAC exhibit APA properties.

Several proteins have been identified as participants in the formation of protein-phospholipid targets for the APAs. Among these proteins are β^2-GpI, prothrombin, protein C and protein S, and annexin-V [12–14,17–22]. The heterogeneity of antibodies in APLS explains the variations in laboratory tests and clinical presentations. Several mechanisms probably are responsible for the variety of clinical and laboratory findings in patients who have APLS. Most probably certain clinical observations and laboratory findings will correlate with specific antibodies to protein phospholipids targets. There reportedly has been a poor correlation between laboratory tests and clinical findings. It also has been suggested that more than one APA probably is present in any given patient [12–14,17–22]. The role of the phospholipids in the phospholipids complex still has not been identified.

LABORATORY DIAGNOSIS OF ANTIPHOSPHOLIPID SYNDROMES

APLS is tested in the laboratory by using both liquid-phase (LAC tests) and the solid-phase ELISA assays (ACAs and other antibody assays). The testing of antibodies to the possible targets of APAs such as β_2-GpI and phosphatidylserine is currently under debate. Many consider the current standard tests for ACA sufficiently sensitive and specific for the diagnosis of APA.

Detection of lupus Anticoagulants

The term "lupus anticoagulant" has caused much confusion. The anticoagulant concept arises because of the prolongation of the phospholipid clotting times that depend on clot-based assays. This prolongation results from LAC's specificity for phospholipids bound to certain proteins [23]. This in vitro phenomenon is manifested as a prolongation in the clotting assays. (The Subcommittee for the International Society on Thrombosis and Haemostasis (ISTH) has tried to change the name but has not been able to achieve consensus on an alternative term, so the term "LAC" remains in use [24,25].) To date, there is no reference standard for LAC testing. LAC is detected by using different clot-based laboratory assays. The ISTH has identified the following criteria for the confirmation of a LAC [25,26].

1. Prolongation of a phospholipids-dependent clotting assay
2. Evidence of an inhibitor demonstrated by mixing studies
3. Confirmation of the phospholipids-dependent nature of the inhibitor
4. Lack of specific inhibition of any coagulation factor

Because LAC is known to be very heterogeneous, it is recommended that all patients suspected of having a LAC be tested using at least two clot-based assays with correction of the abnormal assay by adding excess phospholipid [27].

In the presence of the LAC an abnormality exists in the phospholipids-dependant coagulation reactions including the prothrombin time (PT), the activated partial thromboplastin time (aPTT), and the Russell's viper venom time [28,29]. LAC is not directed against a specific factor but against phospholipids bound to proteins. Up to 15% of LACs may be time- and temperature-dependent when mixing studies are performed [2,3,23]. One-stage assays for factors XII, XI, IX, and VIII may yield low values when the standard dilutions of test plasma are used [29]. Usually further dilution of the test plasma causes the measured level of these factors to approach the normal range, creating a dog-leg curve that is a clue to the presence of an inhibitor. With LAC as an inhibitor, this effect will occur with any of the intrinsic pathway factors assayed. An exception occurs in rare patients who have a decreased concentration of prothrombin resulting from accelerated removal of prothrombin antigen–antibody complexes, as sometimes seen in patients who have systemic lupus. This finding is in keeping with the concept that the antibody is detected to a phospholipid–plasma protein complex.

Multiple LAC assays are currently in use. Before these assays as performed, it is essential that blood specimens be collected in 3.2% sodium citrate tubes and centrifuged to obtain platelet-poor plasma with in 4 hours of blood collection. The platelet count in the platelet-poor plasma should be less than 10,000/μL [3]. If the platelet count is higher, the plasma should be recentrifuged before testing or freezing. Outside laboratories should be advised to double-spin the blood before freezing and shipping to ensure a low platelet count. Residual platelets will provide phospholipids that can neutralize LAC and result in false-negative results.

The available assays are based on the use of reagents that contain low concentrations of phospholipids and therefore are sensitive to the LAC in platelet-poor plasma. Initially, a PT was performed with dilute tissue thromboplastin and a reduced number of platelets in the mixture; however, this method missed IgM inhibitors [30]. A new dilute PT assay has become available that uses a re-lipidated recombinant human tissue factor reagent. Similar to the dilute Russell's viper venom time (dRVVT), this assay incorporates a lower concentration of phospholipids in the screening test and a higher concentration in the confirmatory test. The ratio of these two concentrations is determined, and a cut off is set for the presence of LAC [24,30].

In many patients, an abnormal aPTT is the reason for suspecting a LAC. Such patients probably do not have thrombosis. Therefore it may be reasonable first to do a mixing study to see whether an inhibitor accounts for this abnormal aPTT. If this test shows a factor deficiency, there is little reason to suspect a LAC. On the other hand, if an inhibitor is demonstrated, it is mandatory to determine the nature of the inhibitor or inhibitors because factor VIII inhibitors and LACs occasionally have been reported in the same patient [3]. It is reasonable first to exclude the LAC, because it is found much more commonly. The next step would be to use a platelet-neutralization procedure with the aPTT test and to perform a dRVV test. If the results of these tests are both positive for LAC, it is, as a rule, not necessary to search for an inhibitor of factor VIII or factor IX, but it is mandatory to have a PT test as well as a thrombin time to exclude factor deficiencies and heparin, warfarin, or thrombin inhibitors such as hirudin and argatroban [31].

Zhang and colleagues [32] have proposed that a Staclot LA (Diagnostica Stago, Porsipanny, New Jersey) test be used initially when the LAC is suspected . This is a hexagonal phospholipid-based test that is compared with a non–hexagonal-based aPTT using a commercial reagent from a specific source. This method may be practical when the patient does not have a prolonged aPTT and a hypercoagulable state is suspected, because that study showed the Staclot LA test system to be more sensitive to the than two commercially available aPTT reagents that are known to be LAC sensitive. One disadvantage of this proposed algorithm is reagent cost, which in this case is clearly an important laboratory budget consideration.

It is reasonable to use an algorithm beginning with a dRVVT or a dilute prothrombin time (dPT) as the initial screening, especially when the LAC sensitivity of the reagent is not known. It is reasonable to reserve the Staclot LA as a confirmatory test when the dRVVT and/or the dPT are negative. These algorithms are shown in Fig. 1.

Sensitivity of the aPTT to the presence or absence of the LAC is highly dependent on the reagents used. In the presence of acute-phase reactants, however, the aPTT may not be sensitive to the LAC. Many patients who have thrombosis and LAC have normal aPTT's, even with the newer, allegedly more "sensitive" reagents; thus, the aPTT alone is not a reliable screening test for LACs and should not be used for this purpose [29,33–36]. In the study performed by Zhang and colleagues [32], only 46% of 28 patients who were positive for the LAC showed a positive test using an aPTT-LAC sensitive reagent. When the presence of a LAC is suspected, an additional confirmatory test, preferably the dRVVT, should be performed immediately, regardless of the aPTT.

Another test known as the "platelet neutralization procedure" also has been used to determine the presence of LAC. In this assay platelet-poor plasma from the patient is mixed with platelet membranes, which is the source of phospholipids. In the presence of LAC, the aPTT will be shortened after the addition of the platelet membrane. Several laboratories still use this assay, but it does not have the same sensitivity as some of the newer assays [24,36].

Subsequently, a "modified" Russell's viper venom time was developed in which the venom is diluted to give a "normal" time of 23 to 27 seconds, and the phospholipid then is diluted down to the minimal level that continues to support this range. A prolongation of this system will not correct with a mixture of patient and normal plasma; this system detects both IgG and IgM LACs [35]. The dRVVT assay seems to be one of the most sensitive of all assays for the LAC. Russell's viper venom activates factor Xa. The dilute reagents contain low levels of phospholipids; if the screening test is prolonged and not corrected, the dRVVT confirmatory test should be performed. In the confirmatory assay a higher amount of phospholipids is added, which will neutralize the LAC, if present. In this assay a ratio is derived from the screening and confirmatory assays. Individual laboratory cutoffs should be established to determine the presence of the LAC. At present, the dRVVT is the best test to detect LAC; if this test is prolonged, the presence of a lupus inhibitor can be confirmed by adding phospholipids and noting correction of the prolonged dRVVT [28,29]. Both heparin and warfarin are capable of prolonging the dRVVT.

The kaolin clotting time test also has been modified to assay for the LAC inhibitor. In the kaolin clotting time test, platelet-poor plasma is mixed with varying proportions of test plasma and normal plasma. Kaolin is added, and the time required for clotting is determined [29]. The kaolin clotting time then is plotted against proportions of patients' plasma with normal plasma; an inhibitor is assumed to be present when a small portion of test plasma, in comparison with normal plasma, prolongs the assay. A kaolin aPTT, with rabbit brain phospholipids in a standard and fourfold increased "high" lipid

LABORATORY EVALUATION OF THE ANTIPHOSPHOLIPID SYNDROME 25

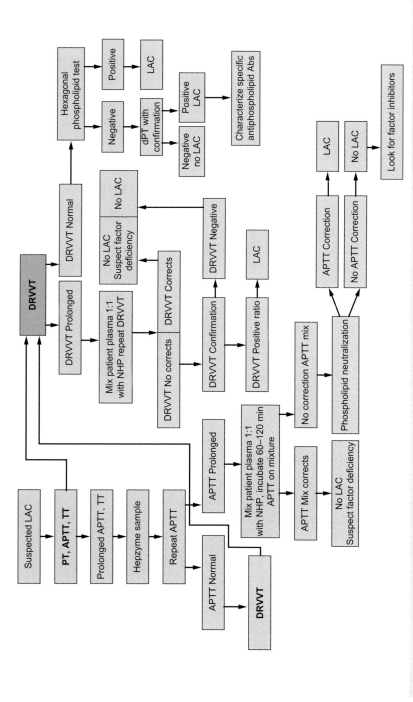

Fig. 1. Initial screening test algorithm. NHP, normal human pooled plasma; TT, thrombin time.

concentration to normalize or "out-inhibit" the abnormal "standard" aPTT, also has been used in diagnosis of the lupus inhibitor [29]. This method is known as the "rabbit brain neutralization procedure"; although it is specific (because of rabbit brain neutralization), it is less sensitive than the dRVVT.

An assay known as the "hexagonal-phase phospholipid neutralization test" also has been used to detect the presence of the LAC. In this assay, the LAC, if present, is neutralized by the hexagonal-phase phosphatidylethanolamine [24]. This test combines all of the ISTH criteria into one assay. Because this assay is based on the aPTT, elevated factor VIII levels may interfere in this assay [24].

As a practical matter, most clinicians and laboratories are asked to evaluate a patient for LAC after the patient has started anticoagulant therapy. Both heparin and warfarin prolong most of the tests mentioned previously, including the most sensitive test, the dRVVT. If the patient is taking warfarin, and the dRVVT is prolonged and then neutralized by appropriate phospholipids, a LAC is confirmed [28,29]. If, however, the patient is taking heparin and the dRVVT is prolonged, the neutralization by platelet-derived phospholipids is not confirmatory, because large amounts of platelet-derived platelet factor IV may inhibit the heparin effect to correct the test. For example, a commercially available platelet extract for the platelet neutralization procedure was found to contain about 100 IU/mL of platelet factor IV, and normal male freeze-thaw platelet extract, commonly prepared for "platelet or phospholipids neutralization procedures" in the clinical laboratory, contains about 95 IU/mL of platelet factor IV. These quantities are sufficient to neutralize heparin and shorten a prolonged clotting test, thereby rendering a false-positive result for LAC in the dRVVT or platelet neutralization procedure [28,29]. As a practical matter, therefore, use of the dRVVT offers the most sensitive assay for detection of a LAC, and neutralization of this test by a non–platelet-derived phospholipids, in particular cephalin, which contains no platelet factor IV, makes this test the most specific as well. In addition, many of the commercial dRVVT reagents have some sort of heparin neutralizer that is effective up to 1.0 U/mL of heparin [36].

More recently, with the introduction of newer drugs such as the thrombin inhibitors, some publications have warned that these drugs might affect the interpretation of testing for LAC. Because these agents are capable of inhibiting thrombin and thrombin generation, they interfere in the formation of fibrinogen to fibrin [32]. In addition, with the development of the new anti-Xa agents, similar caution must be used in interpreting these results [37]. Therefore it is important to screen these patients by using the global PT, aPTT, and thrombin time assays.

Because of the marked heterogeneity of APAs, especially in the secondary APLS, there is a correlation between elevated ACAs and the LAC in secondary antiphospholipid-thrombosis syndromes. LAC and ACAs are two separate entities, however, and usually one occurs without the other being present, especially in the primary antiphospholipid thrombosis syndromes [38]. LAC has a stronger association with binding phospholipids of a hexagonal composition such as phosphatidylcholine, with membrane damage by infection, interleukin-1, or with other mechanisms leading to change from the lamellar to hexagonal form, whereas anticardiolipin antibodies have an affinity to lamellar phospholipids in a bilayer (lamellar) composition [39].

Detection of Anticardiolipin Antibodies

APAs arise as IgM, IgG, or IgA subtypes. They are referred to as "nonspecific inhibitors." Initially these antibodies were thought to bind directly to the phospholipids, but it now is recognized that the target antigens are the proteins that are assembled on the surface of the phospholipids [40]. The most common plasma protein bound to APA is B_2-GpI. Both prothrombin and annexin-V have also been found to bind APAs [13,14,17–19].

The detection of ACAs is straightforward, and there is general agreement that solid-phase ELISA is the method of choice [41–43]. In the past, only IgG and IgA idiotypes were assayed; however, with current recognition that IgM idiotypes, whether primary or secondary (especially drug-induced,) also are associated with thrombosis, most laboratories are, or should be, assaying all three idiotypes. The idiotype distribution of ACAs in patients who have thrombosis is depicted in Box 2. Thus, the appropriate assay for detecting anticardiolipins is solid-phase ELISA, measuring all three idiotypes, IgG, IgA, and IgM [43].

In these assays the microtiter plates are coated with bovine heart cardiolipin and blocked with B_2-GpI. The ACAs in patients bind to the cardiolipin β2-GpI. An enzyme-labeled IgG, IgM, or IgA conjugate is added, and a substrate detects the presence of ACA [3]. The results are given in terms of unit of IgG (GPL), IgM (MPL), or IgA (APL). Each laboratory should establish its own reference limits [3].

Detection of Subtypes of Antiphospholipid Antibodies

When patients experiencing thrombosis or recurrent miscarriage are suspected of harboring APAs and assays for ACAs or LACs are negative, the clinician should suspect discordant subgroups and order assays for anti-B_2-GpI and antibodies to phosphatidylserine, phosphatidylethanolamine, phosphatidylglycerol, phosphatidylinositol, annexin-V, and phosphatidylcholine. These assays are all available by enzyme immunoassay. There is significant discordance between these subgroups and LACs of the three ACA idiotypes; thus they must be tested for in the appropriate clinical situations [44–46].

Box 2: Idiotype/isotype distribution in antiphospholipid syndrome

36% have isolated IgG
17% have isolated IgM
14% have isolated IgA
33% have various admixtures

Box 3: Important antiphospholipid antibodies in thrombosis

Lupus anticoagulant (IgG & IgM)
Anticardiolipin antibodies (IgG, IgA, IgM)
Beta-2-Glycoprotein 1
Hexagonal phospholipid
Subgroups
   Anti-phosphatidylserine (IgG, IgA, IgM)
   Anti-phosphatidylethanolamine (IgG, IgA, IgM)
   Anti-phosphatidylinositol (IgG, IgA, IgM)
   Anti-phosphatidylcholine (IgG, IgA, IgM)
   Anti-phosphatidylglycerol (IgG, IgA, IgM)
   Anti-phosphatidic acid (IgG, IgA, IgM)
   Anti-Annexin-V antibodies (IgG & IgM)

As mentioned previously, discordance will be seen in a significant number of patients. In particular, many patients will have subgroups and APAs (β_2-GpI, anti-phosphatidylserine, anti-phosphatidylcholine, anti-phosphatidylglycerol, anti-phosphatidylinositol, anti-annexin-V antibody, and anti-phosphatidylethanolamine) in the absence of ACAs (IgG, IgA, or IgM) or LAC. Specifically, such findings will be seen in 7% of patients who have antiphospholipid thrombosis syndrome and deep vein thrombosis/pulmonary embolism (type I), in 15% of those who have coronary artery or peripheral arterial thrombosis (type II), in 15% to 24% of those who have cerebrovascular or retinal vascular thrombosis (type III), and in 22% of those who have recurrent miscarriage syndrome (type V). All APAs of importance that have been identified to date are depicted in Box 3. The tests at the top are ordered first, and those at the bottom are ordered if there is clinical suspicion of a subgroup. Fig. 2

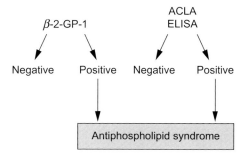

Fig. 2. Laboratory diagnosis of APLS. If these tests are negative, and further testing is clinically indicated, test for subgroup APAs.

depicts an approach to identifying the antibodies present in patients who have APLS.

SUMMARY

APAs are strongly associated with thrombosis and are the most common of the acquired blood protein defects causing thrombosis. Although the precise mechanisms whereby APAs alter hemostasis to induce a hypercoagulable state remain unclear, numerous theories, as previously discussed, have been advanced.

Because the aPTT, including "sensitive systems," is unreliable in patients who have LAC (prolonged in only about 40%–50% of patients) and usually is not prolonged in patients who have ACAs, definitive tests including ELISA for ACA, the dRVVT for LAC, the hexagonal phospholipids neutralization procedure, and B_2-GpI (IgG, IgA, and IgM) should be ordered immediately when APLS is suspected or when patients have otherwise unexplained thrombotic or thromboembolic events. If these tests are negative, in the appropriate clinical setting, subgroups should also be assessed by ELISA. Finally, most patients who have antiphospholipid thrombosis syndrome do not respond to warfarin therapy and, except for those who have retinal vascular thrombosis, may not respond to some types of antiplatelet therapy. Thus it is important to make this diagnosis so that patients can be treated with the most effective therapy for secondary prevention (ie, low molecular weight heparin or unfractionated heparin in most instances and clopidogrel in some instances).

SUMMATION OF THE INTERNATIONAL SOCIETY ON THROMBOSIS AND HAEMOSTASIS SUBCOMMITTEE SESSION IN GENEVA, SWITZERLAND 2007

At the most recent Scientific Subcomittee meeting in Geneva, Switzerland several topics regarding APS were discussed. The following section summarizes this meeting. Topics discussed included the greater frequency of false-positive diagnosis of LAC observed in the elderly population. Awareness of this trend may help the physician and pathologist determine if these patients have a true LAC. Several speakers proposed that a reference preparation or reference plasma for LAC be available through the SSC. Dr. Tripodi from Italy discussed the plans to prepare a lyophilized plasma preparation with an assigned potency and to send preparation out to different laboratories to assess the value of different testing schemes. In addition, there was a suggestion for the standardization of ACA and anti-$β_2$-GpI at the level of the manufacturer. Several presenters discussed the results of various studies assess the clinical significance of LAC and APA to predict patients at risk for developing thrombosis, abortions, and cardiovascular mortality. The following six questions were proposed to the speakers [47]:

1. Would you like to eliminate ACA ELISA from the screening test for APLS?
2. Would you like to eliminate IgM isotype from the ELISA tests for APLS?

3. Do you agree with the Sydney consensus recommendations that a diagnosis of APLS can be made on the basis of testing for ACA alone?
4. Do you agree with the Sydney consensus recommendations that a diagnosis of APLS can be made on the basis of testing for anti-β2-GpI alone?
5. Should the guidelines for the diagnosis of LAC be updated?
6. Would you like to change the laboratory classifications for the diagnosis of APLS?

References

[1] Bick RL, Jakway J, Baker WF. Deep vein thrombosis: prevalence of etiologic factors and results of management in 100 consecutive patients. Semin Thromb Hemost 1992;18: 267–74.
[2] Bick RL, Baker WF. Anticardiolipin antibodies and thrombosis. Hematol Oncol Clin North Am 1992;6:1287–99.
[3] Fritsma GA, Marques MB. Thrombosis risk testing. In: Rodah BF, Fritsma GA, Doig K, editors. Hematology: clinical principles and applications. St. Louis (MO): Saunders Elsevier; 2007. p. 605–28.
[4] Triplett DA. Laboratory diadnosis of lupus anticoagulant. Semin Thromb Hemost 1990;16: 182–92.
[5] Conle CL, Hartmann RC. A hemorrhagic disorder caused by circulating anticoagulants in patients with disseminated lupus erythematosus. J Clin Invest 1952;31:621–2.
[6] Bowie EJW, Thompson JH, Pascuzzi CA, et al. Thrombosis in systemic lupus erythematosus despite circulating anticoagulants. J Lab Clin Med 1963;62:416–30.
[7] Alarcon-Segovia D. Clinical manifestations of the antiphospholipid syndrome. J Rheumatol 1992;18:1916–8.
[8] Triplett DA. Antiphospholipid antibodies and thrombosis. A consequence, coincidence, or cause? Arch Pathol Lab Med 1993;117:78–88.
[9] Harris EN, Gharavi AE, Boey ML. Anticardiolipin antibodies: detection by radioimmunoassays and association with thrombosis in systemic lupus erythematosus. Lancet 1983;2: 1211–4.
[10] Bick RL, Ucar K. Hypercoagulability and thrombosis. Hematol Oncol Clin North Am 1992;6:1421–31.
[11] Triplett DA. Antiphospholipid antibodies. In: Hathway WE, Goodnight SH, editors. Disorders of hemostasis and thrombosis. 2nd edition. New York: McGraw-Hill; 2001. p. 405–19.
[12] Angles-Cano E, Sultan Y, Clauvel JP. Predisposing factors to thrombosis in systemic lupus erythematosus: possible relation to endothelial damage. J Lab Clin Med 1979;94: 317–23.
[13] Nakamura N, Kawasaki C, Shidara Y, et al. Antibody to annexin V has anti-phospholipid and lupus anticoagulant properties. Am J Hematol 1995;49:347–8.
[14] Kaburaki J, Kuwan M, Yamamoto M, et al. Clinical significance of anti-annexin V antibodies in patients with systemic lupus erythematosus. Am J Hematol 1997;54:209–13.
[15] Lie JT. Vasculopathy of the antiphospholipid syndromes revisited: thrombosis is the culprit and vasculitis the consort. Lupus 1966;5:368–71.
[16] Lopez-Pedrera C, Buendia P, Barbarroja N, et al. Antiphospholipid mediated thrombosis: interplay between anticardiolipin antibodies and vascular cells. Clin Appl Thromb Hemost 2006;12:41–5.
[17] McNeil HP, Simpson RJ, Chesterman CN, et al. Antiphospholipid antibodies are directed against a complex antigen that includes a lipid binding inhibitor of coagulation: 2 glycoprotein I (apolipoprotein H). Proc Natl Acad Sci U S A 1990;87:4120–4.

[18] Miesbach W, Matthias T, Scharrer I. Identification of thrombin antibodies in patients with antiphospholipid syndrome. Ann N Y Acad Sci 2005;1050:250–6.
[19] Bertolaccini ML, Hughes GR. Antiphospholipid antibody testing: which are most useful for diagnosis? Rheum Dis Clin North Am 2006;32:455–63.
[20] Roubey AS. Autoantibodies to phospholipid-binding plasma proteins: a new view of lupus anticoagulants and other "antiphospholipid" autoantibodies. Blood 1994;84:2854–67.
[21] Oosting JD, Derksen RHWM, Bobbick IWG, et al. Antiphospholipid antibodies directed against a combination of phospholipids with prothrombin, protein C or protein S. An explanation for their pathogenic mechanism. Blood 1993;81:2618–25.
[22] Matsuda J, Gotoh M, Saith M, et al. Anti-annexin antibody in the sera of patients with habitual fetal loss or pre-eclampsia. Thromb Res 1994;75:105–6.
[23] Teruya J, West AG, Suell MN. Lupus anticoagulant assays: questions answered and to be answered. Arch Pathol Lab Med 2007;131(6):885–9.
[24] Exner T, Triplett DA, Taberner D, et al. Guidelines for testing and revised criteria for lupus anticoagulants. Thromb Haemost 1991;65:320–2.
[25] Brandt JT, Triplett DA, Alving B, et al. Criteria for the diagnosis of lupus anticoagulants, an update on behalf of the subcommittee on lupus anticoagulants/antiphospholipid antibodies of the ISTH. Thromb Haemost 1995;74:1597–603.
[26] Greaves M, Cohen H, Machin SJ, et al. Guidelines on the investigation and management of the antiphospholipid syndrome. Br J Haematol 2000;109:704–15.
[27] Acosta M, Edwards R, Jaffe EI, et al. Practical approach to pediatric patients referred with an abnormal coagulation profile. Arch Pathol Lab Med 2005;129:1011–6.
[28] Bick RL, Baker WF. Antiphospholipid syndrome and thrombosis. Semin Thromb Hemost 1999;25:333–9.
[29] Kunkel L. Acquired circulating anticoagulants. Hematol Oncol Clin North Am 1992;6: 1341–58.
[30] Mackie IJ, Lawie AS, Greenfield RS, et al. A new lupus anticoagulant test based on dilute prothrombin time. Thromb Res 2004;114:673–4.
[31] Genzen JR, Miller JL. Presence of direct thrombin inhibitors can affect the results interpretation of lupus anticoagulant testing. Am J Clin Pathol 2005;124(4):586–93.
[32] Zhang L, Whitis JG, Embry MB, et al. A simplified algorithm for the laboratory detection of lupus anticoagulants. Utilization of two automated integrated tests. Am J Clin Pathol 2005;124:894–901.
[33] Triplett DA, et al. Laboratory evaluation of circulating anticoagulants. In: Bick RL, Bennett RM, Byrnes RK, editors. Hematology: clinical and laboratory practice. Saint Louis (MO): C.V. Mosby Publisher; 1993. p. 1539–48.
[34] Mannucci PM, Canciani MT, Mari D, et al. The varied sensitivity of partial thromboplastin and prothrombin time reagents in the demonstration of the lupus-like inhibitor. Scand J Haematol 1979;22:423–32.
[35] Thiagarajan P, Pengo V, Shapiro SS. The use of the diluted Russel viper venom time for the diagnosis of lupus anticoagulants. Blood 1986;68:869–74.
[36] Teruya J, West AG, Suell MN. Lupus anticoagulant assays. Arch Pathol Lab Med 2007;131: 885–9.
[37] Laux V, Hinder M, et al. Rationale for direct factor Xa inhibitors in acute coronary syndromes. In: Kipshidze NN, Fareed J, Mosses JW, editors. Textbook of international cardiovascular pharmacology. London: Informa Healthcare; 2007. p. 119–26.
[38] Bick RL. The antiphospholipid thrombosis syndromes: a common multidisciplinary medical problem. Clin Appl Thromb Hemost 1997;3:270–83.
[39] Rauch J, Tannenbaum M, Janoff AS. Distinguishing plasma lupus anticoagulants from anti-factor antibodies using hexagonal (II) phase phospholipids. Thromb Haemost 1989;62: 892–6.
[40] Kandiah DA, Sheng YH, Krilis SA. Beta-2 glycoprotein I: target antigen for autoantibodies in the:antiphospholipid symdrome. Lupus 1996;5:381–6.

[41] Falcon CR, Hoffer AM, Forastiero RR, et al. Clinical significance of various ELISA assays for detecting antiphospholipid antibodies. Thromb Haemost 1990;64:21–5.
[42] Rudge AC, Reynolds R, Bolye CC, et al. Measurement of anti-cardiolipin antibodies by an enzyme-linked immunosorbent assay (ELISA): standardization and quantization of results. Clin Exp Immunol 1985;62:738–45.
[43] Reyes H, Dearing L, Shoenfeld Y. Antiphospholipid antibodies: a critique of their heterogeneity and hegemony. Semin Thromb Hemost 1994;20:89–100.
[44] Cabral AR, Amigo MC, Cabiedes J, et al. The antiphospholipid/cofactor syndromes: a primary variant with antibodies to beta-2-glycoprotein-I but no antibodies detectable in standard antiphospholipid assays. Am J Med 1996;101:472–81.
[45] Falcon CR, Hoffer AM, Carreras LO. Antiphosphatidylinositol antibodies as markers of the antiphospholipid syndrome. Thromb Res 1990;63:321–2.
[46] Falcon CR, Hoffer AM, Carreras LO. Evaluation of the clinical and laboratory association of antiphosphatodylethanolamine antibodies. Thromb Res 1990;59:383–8.
[47] Lupus anticoagulant/phospholipid-dependent antibodies 2007 SSC Subcommittee minutes. Avaialable at: http://www.med.unc.edu/isth/SSC/07sscminutes/07luous.htm. Accessed September 3, 2007.

The Clinical Spectrum of Antiphospholipid Syndrome

William F. Baker, Jr, MD, FACP[a,b,c,]*,
Rodger L. Bick, MD, PhD, FACP[d]

[a]David Geffen School of Medicine, Center for Health Sciences, University of California, Los Angeles, Los Angeles, CA, USA
[b]California Clinical Thrombosis Center, 9330 Stockdale Highway, Suite 300, Bakersfield, CA 93311, USA
[c]Thrombosis, Hemostasis and Special Hamatology Clinic, Kern Medical Center, Bakersfield, CA 93305, USA
[d]10455 North Central Expressway, Suite 109-320, Dallas, TX 75231, USA

The antiphospholipid syndrome (APS), first described in 1986 by Hughes, Harris, and Gharavi [1], is an acquired thrombophilic disorder in which autoantibodies are produced to a variety of phospholipids and phospholipid-binding proteins [2,3]. Clinical manifestations range from no symptoms to imminently life-threatening, catastrophic APS (CAPS) (Fig. 1). By definition, from the 1999 Sapporo International Consensus Statement on Preliminary Criteria for the Classification of the Antiphospholipid Syndrome, and from the 2006 International Consensus Statement on an Update of the Classification Criteria for Definite Antiphospholipid Syndrome, a patient with "definite" APS must have persistent high-titer antiphospholipid antibodies (aPL) associated with a history of arterial or venous thrombosis (or both), or recurrent pregnancy morbidity [4,5]. Virtually any organ or organ system may be affected by the consequences of large-vessel or microvessel thrombosis (Box 1). More venous thrombotic events than arterial thrombotic events are observed [2,6]. A radiographic series identified 59% of thrombi as venous, 28% as arterial, and 13% as both arterial and venous [6]. It has generally been reported that the most common presentation of APS is deep vein thrombosis (DVT), occurring in from 29% to 55% of patients on follow-up of 6 years. Of these patients, at least 50% are demonstrated to have concomitant pulmonary embolism (PE) [6–8].

Primary APS has generally been defined as the presence of aPL in patients with idiopathic thrombosis but no evidence of autoimmune disease or other inciting factor, such as infection, malignancy, hemodialysis or drug-induced aPL [9]. The term secondary APS has been used when patients with a wide

*Corresponding author. E-mail address: wbaker@thrombosiscenter.com (W.F. Baker, Jr).

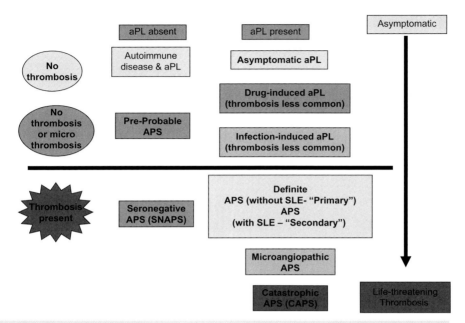

Fig. 1. Clinical spectrum of APS. aPL, antiphospholipid antibodies; SLE, systemic lupus erythematosus.

spectrum of autoimmune disorders (primarily systemic lupus erythematosus [SLE] and rheumatoid arthritis) and thrombosis are also found to have aPL [10,11]. The clinical manifestations of thrombosis are similar, whether the APS is primary or secondary, and the 2006 International Consensus Statement on an Update of the Classification Criteria for Definite Antiphospholipid Syndrome eliminated the "primary" versus "secondary" distinction [2,8,12,13]. In replacing this "primary" versus "secondary" designation, the 2006 criteria designates two subgroups of APS patients—those with and those without the presence of other risk factors for arterial or venous thrombosis [5]. A typical set of clinical manifestations with or without positive serologic tests for aPL, but not qualifying as "definite" APS, has been described as probable APS or pre-APS [14]. A new subset of APS has been proposed, defined as microangiopathic APS [14,15]. The 2006 criteria also identifies patients with typical manifestations of APS but negative aPL serologies (seronegative APS [SNAP]) [16], such as occurs in patients with Sneddon's syndrome (the clinical triad of stroke, livedo reticularis, and hypertension) [17]. Patients may also [12] be found to have aPL in the absence of thrombosis or other manifestations. Patients with infection, malignancy, hemodialysis, and drug-induced aPL are less likely to develop thrombotic events [2,18]. Fig. 1 illustrates these multiple subset individuals with aPL.

Box 1: Clinical manifestations of APS

Thrombosis of large vessels

Neurologic: transient ischemic attack, ischemic stroke, chorea, seizures, dementia, transverse myelitis, encephalopathy, migraines, pseudotumor cerebri, cerebral venous thrombosis, mononeuritis multiplex

Opthalmic: retinal vein and/or artery thrombosis, amaurosis fugax

Cutaneous: superficial phlebitis, leg ulcers, distal ischemia, blue toe syndrome

Cardiac: myocardial infarction, valvular vegetations, intracardiac thrombi, atherosclerosis

Pulmonary: pulmonary emboli, pulmonary hypertension, pulmonary arterial thrombosis, alveolar hemorrhage

Arterial: thrombosis of aorta, thrombosis of large and small arteries

Renal: renal vein/artery thrombosis, renal infarction, acute renal failure, proteinuria, hematuria, nephrotic syndrome

Gastrointestinal: Budd-Chiari syndrome, hepatic infarction, gallbladder infarction, intestinal infarction, splenic infarction, pancreatitis, ascites, esophageal perforation, ischemic colitis

Endocrine: Adrenal infarction or failure, testicular infarction, prostate infarction, pituitary infarction, pituitary failure

Venous thrombosis: Thrombosis in extremities, adrenal thrombosis, hepatic thrombosis, mesenteric thrombosis, thrombosis in splenic veins, vena cava thrombosis

Obstetrical complications: pregnancy loss; intrauterine growth retardation; hemolytic anemia, elevated liver enzymes, and low platelet count (HELLP) syndrome; oligohydraminos; preeclampsia

Hematologic: Thrombocytopenia, hemolytic anemia, hemolytic-uremic syndrome, thrombotic thrombocytopenic purpura

Miscellaneous: perforation of the nasal septum, avascular necrosis of bone

Microvascular thrombosis

Opthalmic: retinitis

Cutaneous: livedo reticularis, superficial gangrene, purpura, ecchymoses, subcutaneous nodules

Cardiac: myocardial infarction, myocardial microthrombi, myocarditis, valvular abnormalities

Pulmonary: acute respiratory distress syndrome, alveolar hemorrhage

Renal: acute renal failure, thrombotic microangiopathy, hypertension

Gastrointestinal: intestinal, hepatic, and splenic infarctions or gangrene

Hematologic: disseminated intravascular coagulation (only in CAPS)

Miscellaneous: microthrombi, microinfarctions

PREVALENCE
In young, apparently healthy control subjects, the prevalence for both lupus anticoagulant and anticardiolipin antibodies (aCL) is about 1% to 5% [19]. The prevalence increases with age, especially in elderly individuals with chronic disease [19]. Although thrombosis may occur in 50% to 70% of patients with aPL and SLE over a 20-year follow-up period, as many as 30% do not develop APS [19]. The Montpellier Antiphospholipid study, which involved 1014 patients admitted to the general medical floor with a variety of diagnoses, found 7.1% with aCL but only 28% of these had clinical features of APS [20]. The risk of thrombosis in patients with APS is estimated to range from 0.5% to 30% [18]. According to analysis of 1000 patients reported by the multicenter Euro-Phospholipid Project, APS syndrome is more common in women than men in about a 5:1 ratio [12]. In patients with SLE, the male/female ratio is even higher (7:1). Female patients also appear to more frequently demonstrate the clinical features of arthritis, livedo reticularis, and migraine, whereas males more often develop myocardial infarction, epilepsy, and lower extremity arterial thrombosis [12]. Although the most common age of onset of the clinical manifestations of APS has a mean of 31 years [12], the disorder may be seen in children and older patients as well. While 85% of patients in the Euro-Phospholipid Project presented between the ages of 15 and 85, onset is uncommon after age 60 [21]. Among patients presenting over the age of 50, males dominated with more strokes and angina pectoris but less livedo reticularis [12].

ASYMPTOMATIC ANTIPHOSPHOLIPID ANTIBODIES
As the precise genesis of aPL is poorly understood. The reason some individuals with no underlying medical disorder develop aPL is also not clear. Why some individuals develop thrombosis and some do not also remains poorly understood. While aPL may be present as a predisposing risk factor, the addition of a triggering risk factor, or "double hit," may be required for the development of thrombosis [2]. Identifiable risk factors for transition from asymptomatic aPL to APS (aPL with thrombosis) include a prior history of thrombosis [22,23], the presence of lupus anticoagulant [24], and an elevated level of aCL IgG [10,25,26]. Various reports suggest that each of these risk factors increase the risk of thrombosis about fivefold [27]. Recent analysis of the Warfarin Anti-Phospholipid Syndrome study by Galli contradicts older studies and confirms that the association between lupus anticoagulant, beta-2-glycoprotein I antibodies (B-2-GP I), antiprothrombin antibodies, and anti–annexin V antibodies with thrombosis is stronger than the association between other aPL and thrombosis [28]. Persistence of aPL over time also progressively increases thrombosis risk [10]. There is no evidence that the presence of risk factors for thrombosis, with the exception of a history of a prior episode of thrombosis, warrants therapeutic anticoagulation in an asymptomatic individual with aPL [2].

As the line between patients with asymptomatic aPL and those with APS is defined by the development of large- or small-vessel thrombosis, or pregnancy loss, it is important to consider the individuals who are asymptomatic as also at risk and deserving of careful clinical surveillance for thrombosis. They are at high risk for the development of venous thrombosis and require meticulous risk assessment and DVT prophylaxis in high-risk clinical circumstances. Similarly, many patients with one thrombophilic disorder are found to have another and the cumulative risk increases with each additional risk factor. As arterial thrombosis is a significant risk for patients with aPL, it is also important to identify patients with other risk factors for arterial thrombosis and to intervene to reduce those risk factors as well. With each additional risk factor for venous or arterial thrombosis, the likelihood increases that an individual with otherwise asymptomatic aPL will transition to primary APS as the result of developing a thrombotic event [2].

PROBABLE ANTIPHOSPHOLIPID SYNDROME

Many patients positive for aPL exhibit clinical features suggesting APS but lack the clinical criteria of vascular thrombosis or pregnancy loss necessary to substantiate a diagnosis of "definite" APS. Such patients have been classified as probable APS or pre-APS [14]. Clinical manifestations include livedo reticularis, chorea, thrombocytopenia, fetal loss, and cardiac valvular lesions [14,29]. The most frequent dermatologic manifestation of APS is livedo reticularis. Some studies have indicated that cutaneous manifestations are the first manifestation of APS in up to 41% of patients with APS [29]. Patients with Sneddon's syndrome who present with livedo reticularis and stroke may have aPL [17] but may also present with the clinical features in the absence of aPL [30]. Livedo reticularis alone may predate APS and the complication of stroke and other types of thrombosis [31]. These patients may also have hypertension, cardiac valvular disorders, epilepsy, and renal artery pathology [14]. Further study is necessary to determine whether patients in the pre-APS category benefit from anticoagulation designed to prevent the later development of vascular thrombosis [14].

SERONEGATIVE ANTIPHOSPHOLIPID SYNDROME

A subset of patients has been identified who exhibit clinical manifestations of APS, without identifiable aPL, lupus anticoagulant, B-2-GP I, antiphospholipid subtype antibodies, or any other recognized aPL on laboratory testing. These individuals are said to have SNAP syndrome [16,30]. Such patients develop idiopathic arterial or venous thrombosis and initial testing for aPL is negative. Repeat testing months later may return positive [30].

DEFINITE ANTIPHOSPHOLIPID SYNDROME

The 1999 Sapporo International Consensus Statement on Preliminary Criteria for the Classification of the Antiphospholipid Syndrome defined patients with primary APS as those with both clinical and laboratory criteria for the diagnosis in the absence of defined connective tissue disease, and patients with secondary APS as those with APS and the presence of connective tissue disease

Box 2: Revised classification criteria for APS

APS is present if at least one of the clinical criteria and one of the laboratory criteria that follow are met.[a]

Clinical criteria

1. Vascular thrombosis[b]

   One or more clinical episodes of arterial, venous[c], or small-vessel thrombosis[d], occurring in any tissue or organ. Thrombosis must be confirmed by objective validated criteria (ie, unequivocal findings of appropriate imaging studies or histopathology). For histopathologic confirmation, thrombosis should be present without significant evidence of inflammation in the vessel wall.

2. Pregnancy morbidity

   (a) One or more unexplained deaths of morphologically normal fetuses at or after the 10th week of gestation, with normal fetal morphology documented by ultrasound or by direct examination of the fetus, or

   (b) One or more premature births of morphologically normal neonates before the 34th week of gestation because of (i) eclampsia or severe preeclampsia defined according to standard definitions or (ii) recognized features of placental insufficiency[e]; or

   (c) Three or more unexplained consecutive spontaneous abortions before the 10th week of gestation, with maternal anatomic or hormonal abnormalities and paternal and maternal chromosomal causes excluded

In studies of populations of patients who have more than one type of pregnancy morbidity, investigators are strongly encouraged to stratify groups of subjects according to a, b, or c above.

Laboratory Criteria[f]

1. Lupus anticoagulant present in plasma on two or more occasions at least 12 weeks apart, detected according to the guidelines of the International Society on Thrombosis and Hemostasis (Scientific Subcommittee on LAs/phospholipid-dependent Antibodies)

2. aCL of IgG and/or IgM isotype in serum or plasma, present in medium or high titer (>40 IgG phospholipid units (GPL) or IgM phospholipid units (MPL), or >99th percentile), on two or more occasions, at least 12 weeks apart, measured by a standardized ELISA

3. Anti–B-2-GP I IgG and/or IgM isotype in serum or plasma (in titer >99th percentile), present on two or more occasions, at least 12 weeks apart, measured by a standardized ELISA, according to recommended procedures

[a]Classification of APS should be avoided if <12 weeks or >5 years separate the positive aPL test and the clinical manifestation.
[b]Coexisting inherited or acquired factors for thrombosis are not reasons for excluding patients from APS trials. However, two subgroups of APS patients should be recognized, according to (a) the presence and (b) the absence of additional risk factors for thrombosis. Indicative (but not exhaustive) of such cases include age (>55 years in men and >65 years in women) and the presence of any of the established risk factors for cardiovascular disease (hypertension, diabetes mellitus, elevated low-density lipoprotein or low high-density lipoprotein cholesterol, cigarette smoking, family history of premature cardiovascular disease, body mass index >30 kg/m^2, microalbunimuria, estimated glomerular filtration rate

<60 mL/min^1), inherited thrombophilias, oral contraceptives, nephrotic syndrome, malignancy, immobilization, and surgery. Thus, patients who fulfill criteria should be stratified according to contributing causes of thrombosis.

^{c}A thrombotic episode in the past could be considered as a clinical criterion, provided that thrombosis is proved by appropriate diagnostic means and that no alternative diagnosis or cause of thrombosis is found.

^{d}Superficial venous thrombosis is not included in the clinical criteria.

^{e}Generally accepted features of placental insufficiency include (i) abnormal or non-reassuring fetal surveillance test(s) (eg, a non-reactive nonstress test suggestive of fetal hypoxemia), (ii) abnormal Doppler flow velocimetry waveform analysis suggestive of fetal hypoxemia (eg, absent end-diastolic flow in the umbilical artery), (iii) oligohydraminos (eg, an amniotic fluid index of 5 cm or less), or (iv) a postnatal birth weight less than the 10th percentile for the gestational age.

^{f}Investigators are strongly advised to classify APS patients in studies into one of the following categories: I, more than one laboratory criteria present (any combination); IIa, lupus anticoagulant present alone; IIb, aCL present alone; IIc, anti–B-2-GP I present alone.

(Box 2). The 2006 International Consensus Statement on an Update of the Classification Criteria for Definite Antiphospholipid Syndrome eliminates this distinction. Criteria used for diagnosis in this article are those of the 2006 Consensus Statement. For a definite diagnosis, patients must have one or more clinical episodes of arterial, venous, or small-vessel thrombosis occurring within any tissue or organ. Thrombosis may include the placenta and result in fetal death or premature birth. Many clinical disorders are associated with the presence of aPL, but not rising to the level of evidence necessary to be included in the 2006 Consensus Statement [5].

Laboratory criteria are well defined and require aCL IgG or IgM or lupus anticoagulant in high titers (>40 IgG phospholipid units [GPL] or IgM phospholipid units [MPL] or >99th percentile), confirmed on repeat testing 12 weeks later [4,5,32]. Not included in the 1999 International Criteria, but included in the 2006 International Criteria are IgG and IgM antibodies to B-2-GP I, which are also highly predictive of risk for thrombosis. Patients may be found to have not only aCL or lupus anticoagulant but also other aPL or combinations [5,12]. Not included in either criteria are antibodies to the antiphospholipid subtypes, anti-prothrombin or anti–annexin V, which have also been linked to risk for thrombotic events [28,33–39]. The report of 1000 patients by Cervera and colleagues [12] concluded that over half of the population with APS has primary APS (53.1%). Patients designated in the pre-2006 literature with primary APS have no clinical or serologic evidence of SLE, rheumatoid arthritis, or any other autoimmune disorder, no history of recent infection, the use of drugs known to trigger aPL, malignancy, or hemodialysis.

The occurrence of clinical manifestations in patients previously designated with primary APS is essentially the same as in patients with the so-called "secondary APS." In the report by Cervera and colleagues [12], the most common were DVT (31.7%), thrombocytopenia (21.9%), stroke (13.1%), superficial thrombophlebitis (9.1%), PE (9.0%), fetal loss (8.3%), transient ischemic attack (7.0%), and hemolytic anemia (6.6%). Typically, the presentation is that of an otherwise healthy and asymptomatic individual presenting with DVT, unexplained thrombocytopenia (platelet count <100,000) or arterial thrombosis (most commonly cerebrovascular). The frequency of idiopathic venous and arterial thrombosis in patients with APS is about equal [8,13]. Both large vessels and small vessels may be involved.

The connective tissue diseases most commonly associated with APS are SLE [40] and rheumatoid arthritis [11]. Other autoimmune disorders reported to be associated with the development of aPL include polymyalgia rheumatica, Behcet's syndrome, scleroderma, Sjogren's syndrome, polyarteritis nodosa, relapsing polychondritis, giant cell arteritis, Takayasu's arteritis, autoimmune hemolytic anemia, Evan's syndrome, and immune thrombocytopenic purpura. The association with SLE and rheumatoid arthritis is well established, while the association with other disorders has relied primarily on case reports [2,41].

As many as 12% to 34% of patients with SLE are identified with aPL [40]. From 12% to 30% have aCL [11] and the prevalence of lupus anticoagulant ranges has been identified in 15% to 34% of SLE patients [40,42]. Of the SLE patients with aPL, 50% to 70% develop APS over the course of a 20-year follow-up. However, as many as 30% of aPL patients fail to demonstrate clinical evidence of thrombotic complications. Cumulative survival of SLE patients with APS (65%) is significantly lower at 15 years than for SLE patients without APS (90%) [43].

Patients with APS and SLE more frequently have arthritis, livedo reticularis, thrombocytopenia, leukopenia, or hemolytic anemia [12,44]. Vascular occlusion of vessels of any size in patients with SLE and APS is due to thrombosis [2]. The histopathologic identification of vascular wall inflammation found in patients with SLE vasculitis is not due to APS.

Cardiac thromboemboli may occur in patients with SLE due to Libman-Sacks verrucous vegetations, which may be responsible for valvular stenosis, insufficiency, and cardiac decompensation. Mitral and aortic valvular lesions are associated with aCL and other manifestations of APS and also correlate with SLE disease duration and disease activity [45]. Patients with aPL may also have a variety of cardiac disorders, independent of the presence of SLE [5].

MICROANGIOPATHIC ANTIPHOSPHOLIPID SYNDROME

Patients with APS may present with a variety of disorders characteristic of microvascular occlusive disease. Such disorders include thrombotic thrombocytopenic purpura (TTP); hemolysis, elevated liver enzymes, and low platelets (HELLP) syndrome; thrombotic microangiopathic hemolytic anemia; and CAPS (Asherson's syndrome). Syndromes may also exhibit overlapping features characteristic of more than one of these conditions. All share the pathologic features of microangiopathy [14].

TTP, characterized by thrombocytopenia, microangiopathic hemolytic anemia, and cerebrovascular ischemia. demonstrates the pathology of microvascular thrombosis typically associated with the presence of large von Willebrand multimers resulting from a deficiency of von Willebrand factor cleaving protease (a disintegrin and metalloproteinase with thrombospondin type 1 motif, 13 [ADAMTS13] deficiency) [46]. Patients are also identified with the concomitant presence of TTP and aPL, as well as TTP, aPL, and SLE [47]. Both primary deficiency of ADAMTS13 [48,49] and ADAMTS13-inhibiting antibodies [50] have been detected in patients with TTP and aPL.

A similar association has been identified in patients with the adult, obstetric form of hemolytic uremic syndrome [51]. Both adults and children with hemolytic uremic syndrome have been identified with renal vascular thrombosis and aPL. A similar pathologic appearance is shared among these syndromes, including the presence of capillary congestion and intracapillary fibrin thrombi. Chronic changes are also observed, with characteristic evidence of chronic hypoperfusion resulting in atrophy, fibrosis, and scarring [51,52].

Pregnant patients with HELLP syndrome and aPL have also been identified [14]. A review of 16 cases of HELLP and aPL suggests that the development of HELLP was promoted by the underlying presence of aPL. Review of the published cases seems to indicate that patients with APS are more likely to have severe HELLP and this is more likely to be associated with preeclampsia or eclampsia [53].

There also are reported cases of severe HELLP who develop clinical and pathologic features of CAPS. Such patients may develop refractory HELLP and systemic complications of microvascular thrombosis [54]. Just as in other patients with CAPS, aggressive therapy involves anticoagulation, intravenous immune globulin, and plasma exchange [14].

DRUG-INDUCED ANTIPHOSPHOLIPID SYNDROME

A variety of medications have been documented to induce the formation of aPL. These have included chlorpromazine, phenytoin, hydralazine, procainamide, fansidar, quinidine, interferon, and cocaine. Most aPL are of the IgM type, present at low levels, and not associated with an increased incidence of thrombosis [55].

INFECTION-ASSOCIATED ANTIPHOSPHOLIPID SYNDROME

A variety of infectious agents trigger the production of aPL [56]. Antibodies induced by infection recognize anionic phospholipid epitopes directly rather than via cofactors such as B-2-GP I. Autoantibodies are more often IgM than IgG. The clinical features typical of APS are less commonly observed with aPL associated with infections [56]. Some infections, however, have been well documented to be associated with the development of aPL and B-2-GP I and are thus more likely to be associated with the subsequent development of thrombosis (leprosy, parvovirus B19, HIV, hepatitus C virus, cytomegalovirus) [56]. Infection may be the triggering factor in as many as 40% of cases of CAPS [57].

MALIGNANCY-ASSOCIATED ANTIPHOSPHOLIPID SYNDROME

It is well known that malignancy is a high-risk condition for venous thrombosis. A variety of solid and hematologic malignancies have been reported to be associated with the presence of aPL. The relationship between malignancy, the development of aPL, and thrombosis is poorly understood [58].

CATASTROPHIC ANTIPHOSPHOLIPID SYNDROME

CAPS, a syndrome of multisystem involvement as a manifestation of APS, was first described by Asherson [59]. The syndrome was coined Asherson's syndrome in 2003 [60]. Occurring in fewer than 1% of APS patients, the syndrome is characterized by multiple small-vessel occlusions leading to multiple organ failure and substantial morbidity and mortality [61]. The syndrome is generally of acute onset and defined by the involvement of at least three different organ systems over a period of days or weeks. Histopathologically, there is evidence of small- and large-vessel occlusions. The striking feature of the syndrome is the presence of an acute microangiopathy, rather than the large-vessel occlusions more typically observed in patients with both primary and secondary APS [57]. Clinical features are the manifestations of organ and tissue ischemia and include renal failure due to renal thrombotic microangiopathy, acute respiratory failure due to adult respiratory distress syndrome, cerebral injury due to microthrombi and microinfarctions, and myocardial failure due to microthrombi [61–63]. The 1998 review by Asherson and colleagues [57,61] of 50 patients (5 from their clinic and 45 by review of the literature), identified as many as 28% of patients with typical features of disseminated intravascular coagulation. Mortality from the largest two reported series, with a total of 130 patients, was as high as 48%. Renal involvement was present in 78%, while 66% had lung involvement, 56% had central nervous system involvement, 50% had cardiac involvement, and 50% had skin involvement [61]. CAPS was more common in females (66%) compared with males (34%). Twenty-eight of the patients (56%) had primary APS, 15 patients (30%) had defined SLE, 6 patients (12%) had "lupuslike" syndrome, and 1 patient (2%) had rheumatoid arthritis. In the review by Asherson and colleagues [61], thrombocytopenia was reported in 34 (68%) patients, and hemolytic anemia in 13 (26%). The detection of autoantibodies was a common finding with lupus anticoagulant (94%), aCL (94%), anti–double-stranded DNA (87% of patients with SLE), antinuclear antibodies (58%), anti-Ro/SS-A (8%), anti–ribonucleic protein (8%), and anti-La/SS-B (2%).

Precipitating factors contributed to the development of CAPS in 11 (22%) patients, with infections in 3, oral contraceptives in 3, surgical procedures in 4 (three minor and one major), withdrawal in anticoagulation in 2, and hysterectomy in 1. A review by Asherson and Cervena in 2003 [56] noted that infection triggered CAPS in as many as 40% of patients with CAPS. An initial thrombosis, felt to be a typical acute thrombosis in a patient with APS, may rapidly evolve into the systemic microangiopathy, described by Kirchens as a "thrombotic storm" [64]. Just as in patients with primary and secondary APS, it may be that a "double or triple hit" is necessary for initiation of the acute systemic microangiopathy [57,63].

International preliminary CAPS classification criteria and treatment guidelines were proposed by the 2002 International Taormina Consensus Statement on Classification and Treatment of CAPS [62]. Criteria for diagnosis include the involvement of three or more organs, systems, and/or tissues (Box 3) [62].

VENOUS THROMBOSIS

Venous thrombosis typically presents with DVT in the lower extremities, observed in 29% to 55% of cases over a follow-up period of less than 6 years [6,7]. As with all cases of venous thromboembolism (VTE), more than half of the patients with symptomatic DVT have asymptomatic PE. When patients

---

Box 3: Preliminary criteria for the classification of CAPS[a]

1. Evidence of involvement of ≥3 organs, systems, and/or tissues[b]
2. Development of manifestations simultaneously or in <1 week
3. Confirmation by histopathology of small-vessel occlusion in at least one organ/tissue[c]
4. Laboratory confirmation of the presence of aPL (lupus anticoagulant and/or aCL an/or anti–B-2-GP I)[d]

Definite CAPS

All four criteria

Probable CAPS

Criteria 2, 3, and 4, plus evidence of involvement of only two organs, systems, and/or tissues

All four criteria, except for the absence of laboratory confirmation of the presence of aPL at least 6 weeks after a first positive result (because of the early death of a patient never tested for aPL before onset of CAPS)[d]

Criteria 1,2, and 4

Criteria 1,3, and 4, plus the development of a third event in >1 week but <1 month, despite anticoagulation treatment

[a]Proposed and accepted during the 10th International Congress on Antiphospholipid Antibodies (aPL), September 2002.
[b]Usually clinical evidence of vessel occlusions, confirmed by imaging techniques when appropriate. Renal involvement is defined by a 50% rise in serum creatinine, severe systemic hypertension (>180/100 mm Hg), and/or proteinuria (>500 mg/24h).
[c]For histopathologic confirmation, significant evidence of thrombosis must be present, although vasculitis may coexist occasionally.
[d]If the patient had not been previously diagnosed as having APS, the laboratory confirmation requires detection of the presence of aPL on two or more occasions at least 6 weeks apart (not necessarily at the time of the event), according to the proposed preliminary criteria for the classification of definite APS.

present with symptoms typical of PE, at least half will not exhibit clinical manifestations of DVT. No particular clinical pattern of venous thrombosis suggests that the patient may have underlying aPL. Unusual sites of venous thrombosis have included the upper extremities, intracranial veins, inferior and superior vena cava, hepatic veins (Budd-Chiari syndrome), portal vein, renal vein, and retinal vein [55,65,66]. Thrombosis of the cerebral veins may present with acute cerebral infarction [67]. The superficial and deep cerebral venous system may be extensively involved. Onset of cerebral venous thrombosis caused by aPL typically presents at a younger age and in a more extensive pattern than onset of cerebral venous thrombosis because of other reasons. Thrombosis of the superior saggital sinus has also been reported [68]. In one series of 40 patients with cerebral venous thrombosis, 3 had aPL and 2 of these 3 also had factor V Leiden mutation [69].

In the setting of idiopathic VTE, laboratory assessment is recommended to search for the presence of underlying thrombophilia. Supporting this is the series of 100 consecutive patients with idiopathic DVT or PE in which 24% were found to have aPL [70]. Testing for aPL is strongly recommended because of the high frequency with which APS is diagnosed [6]. Even in patients with a family history of venous thrombosis, which suggests an underlying inherited thrombophilic disorder, testing for aPL is indicated because many patients with one thrombophilic disorder also have another [71,72]. The clinical manifestations of VTE are the same, whether aPL are present or not. Subsequent to a first episode of VTE, the risk for future venous thrombosis increases significantly. In patients with APS, the risk doubles to at least a 30% risk of recurrence without antithrombotic therapy [23].

ARTERIAL THROMBOSIS

Arterial thromboses are less common than venous thromboses and occur in a variety of settings in patients with primary APS [7,8,73]. Of the 1000 patients in the Euro-Phospholipid Trial, 13.1% presented with stroke, 7% with transient ischemic attack, and 2.8% with acute myocardial infarction [12]. Patients with arterial thrombosis most commonly present with transient ischemic attack or stroke (50%) or myocardial infarction (23%) [7,12,65]. These relatively common arterial occlusive events most suggest APS when they occur in individuals without readily identified risk factors for atherosclerosis. This primarily includes individuals under age 60, without classical risk factors for atherosclerosis (family history, cigarette smoking, hyperlipidemia, hypertension, diabetes mellitus). The presence of aCL is considered to be a risk factor for first stroke [74]. Arterial thrombosis in patients with APS may also involve other large and small vessels, which is somewhat unusual for other thrombophilic disorders or atherosclerotic occlusive disease. These potential arterial thromboses include thromboses of brachial and subclavian arteries, axillary artery (aortic arch syndrome), aorta, iliac, femoral, renal, mesenteric, retinal, and other peripheral arteries [2,7,18]. Clinical manifestations, of course, depend on the caliber and location of the affected artery.

CARDIAC DISORDERS
Arterial occlusion may be either thrombotic or embolic. Premature atherosclerosis appears to be accelerated by the presence of aPL and may predispose to coronary occlusion [75]. Coronary artery thrombosis and embolic occlusion associated with APS results in acute myocardial infarction. Coronary artery graft occlusion [76] and accelerated restenosis of coronary arteries after percutaneous transluminal coronary angioplasty [77] are also more likely in patients with APS. Emboli usually arise from mitral or aortic valve vegetations composed of platelets and fibrin, and may result in cerebrovascular ischemic events [18]. Echocardiography demonstrates at least one valvular abnormality in as many as 63% of APS patients. Many of these are asymptomatic and of unclear clinical significance. However, vegetations of the mitral or aortic valve are observed in 4% of patients [8]. Valvular thickening, vegetations, regurgitation, premature coronary disease, myocardial infarction, dilated diffuse cardiomyopathy, congestive heart failure, pericardial effusion, and pulmonary hypertension have all been observed [78].

NEUROLOGIC DISORDERS
Primary thrombosis and embolic occlusion of cerebral arteries result in cerebral infarction, with clinical manifestations dependent upon the location and caliber of the occluded artery. Most arterial occlusions are of small arteries. Recurrent small strokes may contribute to a picture of multiple-infarct dementia [18]. Typical APS patients with stroke are relatively young and lack other classical risk factors of stroke [79].

Chorea is another clinical disorder that has been strongly linked to the presence of aPL. About 4% of patients with SLE exhibit chorea, which mimics that seen with rheumatic fever (Sydenhan's) or Huntington's chorea. Chorea may predate the development of aPL and may be followed by acute cerebral ischemia. Other central nervous system manifestations associated with aPL include migraine headache, Sneddon's syndrome, seizures, transverse myelitis, Guillain-Barre syndrome, idiopathic intracranial hypertension, cognitive dysfunction, psychosis, and optic neuritis [80].

OBSTETRICAL DISORDERS
As defined in both the 1999 and 2006 International Consensus Statements, fetal demise may be attributed to aPL as unexplained fetal death at or after the 10th week of gestation [4,5]. Premature birth before the 34th week of gestation because of eclampsia or placental insufficiency is also included. Pre-embryonic (<6 weeks' gestation) and embryonic (6 to 9 weeks' gestation) losses are increasingly recognized as an additional complication of aPL. Three or more unexplained consecutive spontaneous abortions before the 10th week of gestation are also among the recognized diagnostic criteria [4,5]. Other complications of pregnancy may also be observed, including eclampsia, intrauterine growth retardation, oligohydraminos, HELLP syndrome, and premature birth. Such patients also demonstrate a high rate of subsequent venous or arterial

thrombosis [81]. Pregnancy complications may occur in patients who are only later found to develop aPL [14,81].

DERMATOLOGIC DISORDERS

Dermatologic manifestations may be the first indication of APS. Histopathologically, the most common feature is noninflammatory vascular thrombosis. Clinically, patients present with livedo reticularis, necrotizing vasculitis, livedoid vasculitis, cutaneous ulcerations and necrosis, erythematous macules, purpura, ecchymoses, painful skin nodules, and subungual splinter hemorrhages. Anetoderma, discoid lupus erythematosus, cutaneous T-cell lymphoma, and disorders similar to Degos and Sneddon's syndrome are also rarely observed [41,82]. Patients with livedo reticularis and APS frequently also have cardiac and cerebral thrombotic events, epilepsy, and migraine headaches [83].

PULMONARY MANIFESTATIONS

The most common pulmonary disorder associated with APS is that of PE. In addition to thromboembolism, in situ thrombosis has been reported. aPL are associated with pulmonary hypertension and, in one study of 38 patients with precapillary pulmonary hypertension, 30% were found to have aPL [84]. Refractory noninflammatory pulmonary vasculopathy characterized by microvascular thrombosis may present primarily or in association with CAPS [41].

GASTROINTESTINAL DISORDERS

Thrombosis of the hepatic veins as a manifestation of APS results in Budd-Chiari syndrome. Mesenteric and portal venous thrombosis in APS are well described. Other manifestations of large- and small-vessel thrombosis include hepatic infarction, pancreatitis, esophageal necrosis, intestinal ischemia and infarction, colonic ulceration, acalculous cholecystitis with gallbladder necrosis, and giant gastric ulceration [18,41].

RENAL MANIFESTATIONS

The primary renal manifestations of APS are associated with thrombotic microangiopathy, designated as aPL-associated nephropathy [5,85]. Other complications may include renal vein thrombosis, renal infarction, renal artery stenosis, and allograft vascular thrombosis [86].

RETINAL DISORDERS

Venous and arterial thrombosis of the retinal vasculature is a well-recognized manifestation of APS. Presentation strongly suggestive of the presence of aPL includes the diffuse occlusion of retinal arteries, veins, or both, and neovascularization at the time of presentation. Other opthalmic manifestations included optic neuropathy and cilioretinal artery occlusion [87].

MISCELLANEOUS MANIFESTATIONS
A wide variety of clinical disorders have been reported in association with APS. Less common but important are adrenal hemorrhage, bone marrow necrosis (especially in CAPS), and sudden acute sensorineural hearing loss [18].

HEMATOLOGIC DISORDERS
Thrombocytopenia (platelet count <100,000) [12] is present in from 20% to 40% of patients with APS and is usually mild [88,89]. Severe thrombocytopenia is most often seen in patients with CAPS and those with concomitant disseminated intravascular anticoagulation or TTP [14]. The association of aPL with autoimmune thrombocytopenic purpura has been recognized since the 1985 report by Harris and colleagues [90] and has more recently been reported to be present in as many as 38% of patients [91]. Follow-up has documented thrombosis in 60% of the patients with aPL and only 2.3% of those without aPL [91,92]. To clarify the significance of thrombocytopenia in patients with aPL, patients are designated as having aPL-associated thrombocytopenia if there is coexistence of aPL laboratory criteria with thrombocytopenia (platelet count <100,000) confirmed at least twice, 12 weeks apart and exclusion of patients with TTP, disseminated intravascular coagulation, pseudothrombocytopenia, or heparin-induced thrombocytopenia [5].

BLEEDING
Patients with APS rarely develop severe bleeding. Hemorrhage may result from a concurrent coagulopathy or disseminated intravascular coagulation, as may be observed in patients with CAPS. Most cases of severe bleeding solely attributable to APS are the result of severe, acquired hypo-prothrombinemia [93]. Prolongation of the prothrombin time and activated partial thromboplastin time may be attributed to the presence of lupus anticoagulant and the severity of prothrombin deficiency not appreciated. A specific assay for prothrombin must be obtained for diagnosis. Other disorders that are linked to aPL and that predispose to bleeding rather than thrombosis, include acquired thrombocytopathies, thrombocytopenia, and acquired inhibitors to coagulation factors [41].

CHILDREN WITH ANTIPHOSPHOLIPID SYNDROME
Children (2.8% in the Euro-Phospholipid cohort) have more commonly presented with chorea and internal jugular thrombosis than is the case in adults [12]. A variety of presentations have been reported in children, including DVT, PE, cerebral stroke, myocardial infarction, and peripheral arterial occlusion [94,95]. An increased incidence of APS has been observed in children with stroke and migraine headaches [96]. Children with lupus anticoagulant more commonly present with venous thrombosis and arterial thrombosis in those with aCL [97].

SUMMARY

APS is a disorder characterized by a wide variety of clinical manifestations. Virtually any organ system or tissue may be affected by the consequences of large- or small-vessel thrombosis. There is a broad spectrum of disease among individuals with aPL, from asymptomatic to imminently life-threatening CAPS. Patients may exhibit clinical features suggesting APS but not fulfill the International Criteria for a "definite" diagnosis. SNAPS patients demonstrate typical idiopathic thromboses but aPL are not initially detected. Patients defined with definite APS demonstrate nearly identical sites of venous and arterial thrombosis, regardless of the presence or absence of SLE. Microangiopathic APS may present with isolated tissue and organ injury or as the overwhelming "thrombotic storm" observed in CAPS.

References

[1] Hughes G, Harris EN, Gharavi A. The anticardiolipin syndrome. J Rheumatol 1986;13:486–9.
[2] Levine JS, Branch DW, Rauch J. The antiphospholipid syndrome. N Engl J Med 2002;346(10):752–63.
[3] Roubey RAS. Immunology of the antiphospholipid antibody syndrome. Arthritis Rheum 1996;39:1444–54.
[4] Wilson W, Gharavi A, Koike T, et al. International consensus statement on preliminary classification criteria for definite antiphospholipid syndrome: report of an international workshop. Arthritis Rheum 1999;42:1309–11.
[5] Miyakis S. International consensus statement on an update of the classification criteria for definite antiphospholipid syndrome (APS). J Thromb Haemost 2006;4:295–306.
[6] Provenzale JM, Ortel T, Allen N. Systemic thrombosis in patients with antiphospholipid syndrome: lesion distribution and imaging findings. Am J Roentgenol 1998;170:285–90.
[7] Asherson R, Khamashta M, Ordi-Rios J, et al. The "primary" antiphospholipid syndrome: major clinical and serological features. Medicine (Baltimore) 1989;68:366–74.
[8] Vianna JL, Khamashta M, Ordi J, et al. Comparison of the primary and secondary antiphospholipid syndrome: a European multicenter study of 114 patients. Am J Med 1994;96:3–9.
[9] Piette JC, Wechsler B, Frances C, et al. Exclusion criteria for primary antiphospholipid syndrome. J Rheumatol 1993;20:1802–4.
[10] Alarcon-Segovia D, Deleze M, O CV, et al. Antiphospholipid antibodies and the antiphospholipid syndrome in systemic lupus erythematosus: a prospective analysis of 500 consecutive patients. Medicine (Baltimore) 1989;68:353–65.
[11] Merkel PA, Chang Y, Pierangeli SS, et al. The prevalence and clinical associations of anticardiolipin antibodies in a large inception cohort of patients with connective tissue diseases. Am J Med 1996;101(6):576–83.
[12] Cervera R, Piette JC, Font J, et al. Antiphospholipid syndrome: clinical and immunologic manifestations and patterns of disease expression in a cohort of 1,000 patients. Arthritis Rheum 2002;46:1019–27.
[13] Krnic B, O'Connor C, Looney S, et al. A retrospective review of 61 patients with antiphospholipid syndrome. Analysis of factors influencing recurrent thrombosis. Arch Intern Med 1997;157:2101–8.
[14] Asherson RA. New subsets of the antiphospholipid syndrome in 2006: "PRE-APS" (probable APS) and microangiopathic antiphospholipid syndromes ("MAPS"). Autoimmun Rev 2006;6(2):76–80.
[15] Schofield Y. Systemic antiphospholipid syndrome. Lupus 2003;12:497–8.
[16] Hughes GR, Khamashta MA. Seronegative antiphospholipid syndrome. Ann Rheum Dis 2003;62(12):1127.

[17] Lotz BP, Schutte CM, Colin PF, et al. Sneddon's syndrome with anticardiolipin antibodies—complications and treatment. S Afr Med J 1993;83(9):663–4.
[18] Gezer S. Antiphospholipid syndrome. Dis Mon 2003;49(12):696–741.
[19] Petri M. Epidemiology of the antiphospholipid antibody syndrome. J Autoimmun 2000;15(2):145–51.
[20] Schved J, Dupuy-Fons C, Biron C, et al. A prospective epidemiological study on the occurrence of antiphospholipid antibody: the Montpellier Antiphospholipid (MAP) study. Hemostasis 1994;24:175–82.
[21] Piette JC, Cacoub P. Antiphospholipid syndrome in the elderly: caution [editorial]. Circulation 1998;97:2195–6.
[22] Finazzi G, Brancaccio V, Moia M, et al. Natural history and risk factors for thrombosis in 360 patients with antiphospholipid antibodies: a four-year prospective study from the Italian Registry. Am J Med 1996;100:530–6.
[23] Schulman S, Svenungsson E, Granqvist S. Group DoAS. Anticardiolipin antibodies predict early recurrence of thromboembolism and death among patients with venous thromboembolism following anticoagulant therapy. Am J Med 1998;104:332–8.
[24] Wahl D, Guillemin F, de Maistre E, et al. Risk for venous thrombosis related to antiphospholipid antibodies in systemic lupus erythematosus—a meta-analysis. Lupus 1997;6:467–73.
[25] Varrala O, Manttari M, Manninen V, et al. Anti-cardiolipin antibodies and risk of myocardial infarction in a prospective cohort of middle-aged men. Circulation 1995;91:23–7.
[26] Levine SR, Salowich-Palm L, Sawaya KL, et al. IgG anticardiolipin antibody titer >40 GPL and the risk of subsequent thrombo-occlusive events and death. A prospective cohort study. Stroke 1997;28(9):1660–5.
[27] Khamashta M, Cuadrado M, Mujic F, et al. The management of thrombosis in the antiphospholipid-antibody syndrome. N Engl J Med 1995;332:993–7.
[28] Galli M, Borrelli G, Jacobsen EM, et al. Clinical significance of different antiphospholipid antibodies in the WAPS (Warfarin in the Anti-Phospholipid Syndrome) study. Blood 2007;110(4):1178–83.
[29] Asherson R, Mayou S, Merry P, et al. The spectrum of livedo reticularis and anticardiolipin antibodies. J Dermatol 1989;120:215–21.
[30] Miret C, Cervera R, Reverter JC, et al. Antiphospholipid syndrome without antiphospholipid antibodies at the time of the thrombotic event: transient "seronegative" antiphospholipid syndrome? Clin Exp Rheumatol 1997;15:541–4.
[31] Tourbach A, Piette JC, Iba-zizzen M, et al. The natural course of cerebral lesions in Sneddon's syndrome. Arch Neurol 1997;54:54–60.
[32] Brandt J, Triplett DA, Alving B, et al. Criteria for the diagnosis of lupus anticoagulants: an update. Thromb Haemost 1995;74:1185–90.
[33] Pengo V, Biasiolo A, Brocco T, et al. Autoantibodies to phospholipid-binding plasma proteins in patients with thrombosis and phospholipid-reactive antibodies. Thromb Haemost 1996;75:721–4.
[34] Roubey R, Harper M, Eisenberg R, et al. "Anticardiolipin" autoantibodies recognize beta 2-glycoprotein I in the absence of phospholipid. Importance of Ag density and bivalent binding. J Immunol 1995;154:954–60.
[35] Galli M, Comfurius P, Barbui T, et al. Anticoagulant activity of B2-glycoprotein-I is potentiated by a distinct subgroup of anticardiolipin antibodies. Thromb Haemost 1992;68:297–300.
[36] Viard J-P, Amoura Z, Bach J-F. Association of anti-B2 glycoprotein-I antibodies with lupus-type circulating anticoagulant and thrombosis in systemic lupus erythematosus. Am J Med 1992;93:181–6.
[37] Meroni PL, Ronda N, De Angelis V, et al. Role of anti-beta2 glycoprotein I antibodies in antiphospholipid syndrome: In vitro and in vivo studies. Clin Rev Allergy Immunol 2007;32(1):67–74.

[38] Parkpian V, Verasertniyom O, Vanichapuntu M, et al. Specificity and sensitivity of anti-beta(2)-glycoprotein I as compared with anticardiolipin antibody and lupus anticoagulant in Thai systemic lupus erythematosus patients with clinical features of antiphospholipid syndrome. Clin Rheumatol Mar 2, 2007.
[39] Bas de Laat H, Derksen RH, de Groot PG. beta2-glycoprotein I, the playmaker of the antiphospholipid syndrome. Clin Immunol 2004;112(2):161–8.
[40] Cervera R, Khamashta MA, Font J, et al. Systemic lupus erythematosus: clinical and immunologic patterns of disease expression in a cohort of 1,000 patients. The European Working Party on Systemic Lupus Erythematosus. Medicine (Baltimore) 1993;72(2):113–24.
[41] Rand JH. The antiphospholipid syndrome. In: Beutler E, editor. Williams hematology. 6th edition. New York: McGraw-Hill; 2001. p. 1715–33.
[42] Love P, Santoro S. Antiphospholipid antibodies: anticardiolipin and the lupus anticoagulant in systemic lupus erythematosus (SLE) and in non-SLE disorders: prevalence and clinical significance. Ann Intern Med 1990;112:682–98.
[43] Ruiz-Irastorza G, Egurbide MV, Ugalde J, et al. High impact of antiphospholipid syndrome on irreversible organ damage and survival of patients with systemic lupus erythematosus. Arch Intern Med 2004;164(1):77–82.
[44] Arnout J, Jankowski M. Antiphospholipid syndrome. Hematol J 2004;(5 Suppl 3):S1–5.
[45] Moyssakis I, Tektonidou M, Vasilliou V, et al. Libman-Sacks endocarditis in systemic lupus erythematosus: prevalence, associations and evolution. Am J Med 2007;120: 636–42.
[46] Lammle B, Kremer Hovinga JA, Alberio L. Thrombotic thrombocytopenic purpura. J Thromb Haemost 2005;3(8):1663–75.
[47] Musa M, Nounou R, Sahovic E, et al. Fulminant thrombotic thrombocytopenic purpura in two patients with systemic lupus erythematosus and phospholipid autoantibodies. Eur J Haematol 2000;64:433–5.
[48] Matsuda J, Sanaka T, Gonichi K, et al. Occurrence of thrombotic thrombocytopenic purpura in a systemic lupus patient with antiphospholipid antibodies in association with a decreased activity of von Willebrand-factor cleaving protease. Lupus 2002;11:463–4.
[49] Amoura Z, Costedoat-Chalimeau N, Veyradier A, et al. Thrombotic thrombocytopenic purpura with ADAMTS-13 deficiency in two patients with primary antiphospholipid syndrome. Arthritis Rheum 2004;50:3260–4.
[50] Rieger M, Mannucci PM, Kremer Hovinga JA, et al. ADAMTS-13 autoantibodies in patients with thrombotic microangiopathies and other diseases. Blood 2005;106:1262–7.
[51] Kniaz D, Eisenberg R, Elrad H, et al. Post-partum hemolytic-uremic syndrome associated with antiphospholipid antibodies. Am J Nephrol 1992;12:126–33.
[52] Ardiles L, Olavarria F, Elgueta M, et al. Anticardiolipin antibodies in classic pediatric hemolytic-uremic syndrome: possible pathogenetic role. Nephron 1998;78:278–83.
[53] Le Thi Thuong D, Tieulie N, Costedoat-Chalimeau N, et al. The HELLP syndrome in the antiphospholipid syndrome: retrospective study of 16 cases in 15 women. Ann Rheum Dis 2005;64:273–8.
[54] Koenig M, Roy M, Baccot S, et al. Thrombotic microangiopathy with liver, gut and bone infarction (catastrophic antiphospholipid syndrome) associated with HELLP syndrome. Clin Rheumatol 2005;2:166–8.
[55] Bick R, Baker W. Anticardiolipin antibodies and thrombosis. Hematol Oncol Clin North Am 1992;6:1287–99.
[56] Asherson R, Cervera R. Antiphospholipid antibodies and infections. Ann Rheum Dis 2003;62:388–93.
[57] Asherson R, Cervera R, Piette JC. Catastrophic antiphospholipid syndrome: clues to the pathogenesis from a series of 80 patients. Medicine (Baltimore) 2001;80:355–77.
[58] Zuckerman E, Toubi E, Golan T, et al. Increased thromboembolic incidence in anti-cardiolipin-positive patients with malignancy. Br J Cancer 1995;72:447–51.

[59] Asherson R. The catastrophic antiphospholipid syndrome [editorial]. J Rheumatol 1992;19: 508–12.
[60] Piette JC, Cervera R, Levy RA, et al. The catastrophic antiphospholipid syndrome-Asherson's syndrome. Ann Med Interne (Paris) 2003;154:195–6.
[61] Asherson RA, Cervera R, Piette JC, et al. Catastrophic antiphospholipid syndrome. Clinical and laboratory features of 50 patients. Medicine (Baltimore) 1998;77(3):195–207.
[62] Asherson RA. Catastrophic antiphospholipid syndrome: international consensus statement on classification criteria and treatment guidelines. Lupus 2003;12:530–4.
[63] Erkan D, Cervera R, Asherson RA. Catastrophic antiphospholipid syndrome: Where do we stand? Arthritis Rheum 2003;48(12):3320–7.
[64] Kirchens C. Thrombotic storm: when thrombosis begets thrombosis. Am J Med 1998;104: 381–5.
[65] Bick R, Baker W. Antiphospholipid syndrome and thrombosis. Semin Thromb Hemost 1999;25:333–50.
[66] Provenzale JM. Anatomic distribution of venous thrombosis in patients with antiphopholipid antibody: image findings. AJR Am J Roentgenol 1995;165:365–8.
[67] Carhuapoma J, Mitsias P, Levine SR. Cerebral venous thrombosis and anticardiolipin antibodies. Stroke 1997;28:2363–9.
[68] Nagai S, Horie Y, Akai T, et al. Superior saggital sinus thrombosis associated with primary antiphospholipid syndrome—case report. Neurol Med Chir (Tokyo) 1998;38:34–9.
[69] Deschiens M, Conrad J, Horellou M, et al. Coagulation studies, factor V Leiden, and anticardiolipin antibodies in 40 cases of cerebral venous thrombosis. Stroke 1996;27:1724–9.
[70] Bick R, Jakway J, Baker W. Deep vein thrombosis: prevalence of etiologic factors and results of management in 100 consecutive patients. Semin Thromb Hemost 1992;18:267–74.
[71] Montaruli B, Borchiellini A, Tamponi G, et al. Factor V Arg-Gln mutation in patients with antiphospholipid antibodies. Lupus 1996;5:303–6.
[72] Schutt M, Kluter H, Hagedorn G, et al. Familial coexistence of primary antiphospholipid syndrome and factor V Leiden. Lupus 1998;7:176–82.
[73] Alarcon-Segovia D, Perez-Vasquez M, Villa A, et al. Preliminary classification criteria for the antiphospholipid syndrome with systemic lupus erythematosus. Semin Arthritis Rheum 1992;21:275–86.
[74] Group APASS. Anticardiolipin antibodies and the risk of recurrent thrombo-occlusive events and death. Neurology 1997;48:91–4.
[75] Ames PR, Margarita A, Sokoll KB, et al. Premature atherosclerosis in primary antiphospholipid syndrome: preliminary data. Ann Rheum Dis 2005;64(2):315–7.
[76] Morton K, Gavaghan S, Kirilis S, et al. Coronary artery bypass graft failure: an autoimmune phenomenon? Lancet 1986;2:1353–7.
[77] Ludia C, Domenico P, Monia C, et al. Antiphospholipid antibodies: a new risk factor for restenosis after percutaneous transluminal coronary angioplasty? Autoimmunity 1998;27:141–8.
[78] Kaplan S, Chartash E, Pizzarello R, et al. Cardiac manifestations of the antiphospholipid syndrome. Am Heart J 1992;124:1331–8.
[79] Brey RL. Management of the neurological manifestations of APS—What do the trials tell us? Thromb Res 2004;114(5–6):489–99.
[80] Sanna G, Bertolaccini ML, Hughes GR. Hughes syndrome, the antiphospholipid syndrome: a new chapter in neurology. Ann N Y Acad Sci 2005;1051:465–86.
[81] Carp HJA. Antiphospholipid syndrome in pregnancy. Curr Opin Obstet Gynecol 2004;16: 129–35.
[82] Gibson G, Su W, Pittelkow M. Antiphospholipid syndrome and the skin. J Am Acad Dermatol 1997;36:970–82.
[83] Toubi E, Krause I, Fraser A, et al. Livedo reticularis as a marker for predicting multisystem thrombosis in antiphospholipid syndrome. Clin Exp Rheumatol 2005;23:499–504.

[84] Karmochkine, Cacoub P, Dorent R, et al. High prevalence of antiphospholipid antibodies in precapillary pulmonary hypertension. J Rheumatol 1996;23:286–90.
[85] Nochy D, Daugas E, Droz D, et al. The intrarenal vascular lesions associated with primary antiphospholipid syndrome. J Am Soc Nephrol 1999;10(3):507–18.
[86] Nzerue C, Hewan-Lowe K, Pierangeli S, et al. "Black swan in the kidney:" renal involvement in the antiphospholipid antibody syndrome. Kidney Int 2002;62:733–44.
[87] Dunn J, Noorily S, Petri M, et al. Antiphospholipid antibodies and retinal vascular disease. Lupus 1996;5:313–22.
[88] Galli M, Finazzi G, Barbui T. Thrombocytopenia in the antiphospholipid syndrome: pathophysiology, clinical relevance and treatment. Ann Med Interne (Paris) 1996;147(Suppl 1): 24–7.
[89] Cuadrado M, Mujic F, Munoz E, et al. Thrombocytopenia in the antiphospholipid syndrome. Ann Rheum Dis 1997;56:194–6.
[90] Harris EN, Gharavi A, U H, et al. Anticardiolipin antibodies in autoimmune thrombocytopenic purpura. Br J Haematol 1985;59:231–4.
[91] Diz-Kucukkaya R, Hachihanafioglu A, Yenerei E, et al. Antiphospholipid antibodies and antiphospholipid syndrome in patients presenting with immune thrombocytopenic purpura: a prospective cohort study. Blood 2001;98:1760–4.
[92] Atsumi T, Furukawa S, Amengual O, et al. Antiphospholipid antibody associated thrombocytopenia. Lupus 2005;14:499–504.
[93] Vivaldi P, Rossetti G, Galli M, et al. Severe bleeding due to acquired hypoprothrombinemia-lupus anticoagulant syndrome. Haemotologica 1997;82:345–7.
[94] Campos LMA. Antiphospholipid antibodies and antiphospholipid syndrome in 57 children and adolescents with systemic lupus erythematosus. Lupus 2003;12:820–6.
[95] Gattorno M, Falcini F, Ravelli A, et al. Outcome of primary antiphospholipid syndrome in childhood. Lupus 2003;12(6):449–53.
[96] Pilarska E, Lemka M, Bakowska A. Prothrombotic risk factors in ischemic stroke and migraine in children. Acta Neurol Scand 2006;114(1):13–6.
[97] Barlas S, Tansel T. Antiphospholipid syndrome in a child: an insight into the pathology, identification, and means of cure. J Pediatr Surg 2004;39(8):1280–2.

Antiphospholipid Antibody Syndrome and Autoimmune Diseases

Rochella A. Ostrowski, MD[a,*], John A. Robinson, MD[b]

[a]Division of Rheumatology, Department of Medicine, Loyola University Medical Center, 2160 South First Avenue, Building 54, Room 119, Maywood, IL 60153, USA
[b]Division of Rheumatology, Department of Medicine, Loyola University Medical Center, 2160 South First Avenue, Building 54, Room 113, Maywood, IL 60153, USA

For several decades, clinical distinctions have been drawn between patients who have antiphospholipid antibody syndrome (APS) and no other defining disease and patients who have an autoimmune disease and APS. The lack of insight into the mechanisms of APS has prompted the identification of three clinical phenotypes: primary APS (PAPS), secondary APS, and catastrophic APS (CAPS).

Two other groups of diverse patients, those with acute and chronic infectious diseases [1] and the elderly [2], can also have phospholipid autoantibody profiles that might suggest the diagnosis of APS to the unwary clinician.

As the understanding of the immunoregulation of autoantibody production increases, appreciation of the extreme polymorphism of immune responses that dictate a wide spectrum of clinical disease expression grows, and the critical role of β2 glycoprotein I (β2GPI) antibodies is confirmed in the clinical expression of the hypercoagulable state, the value of segregating patients into clinical subgroups [3] has become questionable.

APS associated with autoimmune disease is often called secondary APS. The former descriptor is better than the latter because the term "secondary" implies that the primary autoimmune disease is causally linked to the presence of the secondary APS, which may be misleading because the fundamental thrombotic mechanism or mechanisms of primary APS and secondary APS are likely the same.

A large body of literature confirms that distinctions between PAPS and so-called "secondary APS" can be difficult to make, especially in the case of systemic lupus erythematosus (SLE) but also in rheumatoid arthritis (RA) and other rheumatologic diseases.

Classifying APS based on clinical expression may not be worth the time and effort and may increase the risk for unnecessary treatment of an erroneous diagnosis based on the epiphenomenon of reactive or immunosenescent

*Corresponding author. E-mail address: rostrowski@lumc.edu (R.A. Ostrowski).

0889-8588/08/$ – see front matter © 2008 Elsevier Inc. All rights reserved.
doi:10.1016/j.hoc.2007.10.003 hemonc.theclinics.com

autoantibody formation. The absence of a clear understanding of the specific factors that collaborate to cause thrombosis and fetal loss in APS confronts the clinician with the difficult task of separating the serious from the benign. This dilemma is likely to be resolved in the future but, until that time, a discussion of the prevalence and implications of APS in autoimmune diseases can provide a perspective of the magnitude of the problem. For ease of discussion in the remainder of this article, antiphospholipid antibodies (aPL) refer to any and all antibodies that have been implicated in APS, including anticardiolipin antibodies (aCL), lupus anticoagulant (LAC), and anti-β2GPI antibodies. Specific types of aPL are cited when deemed relevant to the discussion at hand.

ANTIPHOSPHOLIPID ANTIBODY SYNDROME AND AUTOIMMUNE DISEASE: SYSTEMIC LUPUS ERYTHEMATOSUS

SLE exemplifies the difficulty of clinically distinguishing between PAPS and an autoimmune disease associated with aPL. Comparing the diagnostic criteria for APS and the American College of Rheumatology revised criteria for SLE reveal many overlapping features between PAPS and lupus. These include proteinuria, pleuritis, thrombocytopenia, hemolytic anemia, and seizures [4]. The American College of Rheumatology criteria even include the presence of an aPL, usually with anticardiolipin specificity, as a valid criterion for the diagnosis of SLE. Conversely, the high incidence of APS in SLE has led to many APS patients being erroneously diagnosed with SLE on a guilt-by-association basis. Although it is true that antinuclear antibodies detected by routine screening methods are common in PAPS, SLE-specific antibodies like anti-Smith or anti–double-stranded DNA are almost never present [5,6]. The differentiation between PAPS and SLE is not just an academic diagnostic exercise because their treatment and prognosis are significantly different.

Arbitrary inclusion criteria to distinguish between PAPS and SLE co-occurring with APS (SLE/APS) have been proposed but have not been widely tested for their power to differentiate [7]. The definite presence of APS is determined by two or more clinical manifestations such as recurrent fetal loss, venous thrombosis, arterial occlusion, leg ulcer, livedo reticularis, hemolytic anemia, or thrombocytopenia coupled with a high level of IgG or IgM aPL defined as more than five standard deviations from the normal mean of the assay being used. Probable presence of APS in SLE requires one of the clinical manifestations and a high-titer aPL or two or more clinical manifestations and an IgG or IgM aPL between two and five standard deviations from the normal mean of the assay being used. Exclusion criteria with similar limitations have also been proposed [8]. Experienced rheumatologists and hematologists have little difficulty deciding whether a patient has PAPS or APS and SLE. Moreover, the clinical usefulness of differentiating between PAPS and SLE/APS may be moot because the treatment of the APS component is similar.

Another clinical question that often arises in regard to PAPS is whether it can progress over time to SLE/APS. Literature reviews conclude that if SLE does eventually occur in patients who have PAPS [9], it is a rare event, but the duration of follow-up of patients who had PAPS was relatively short and the true incidence may be underestimated [10].

SLE is a commonly reported autoimmune disease associated with APS [11,12]. A wide range of aPL, usually aCL, has been found in SLE. Frequencies that range from 16% to 55% [13–16] have been reported but their significance cannot be assessed because different and outdated criteria for the diagnosis of SLE, and different aPL assays in time, method, and interpretation have been used. The lack of inclusion of β2GPI antibodies in many studies renders aPL frequencies of little value in understanding APS in the context of SLE [9]. A closer look at the frequency of aCL and β2GPI antibody isotypes, epitope specificity, and LAC in SLE/APS reveals that the anti-β2GPI antibody was common, much more frequent in Caucasians, and rarely found in patients who do not have aCL or LAC. More significantly, anti-β2GPI antibodies that remained positive for at least 3 months were associated with arterial and venous thrombosis but not pregnancy loss [16]. The latter study also reinforced the clinical notion that the significance of the IgA isotype of anti-β2GPI remains an enigma. IgA antibodies of any aPL specificity have not been convincingly shown to have any relevance in either PAPS or SLE/APS.

Some clinicians advocate routine screening of SLE patients who have APS antibody panels [17]. This practice has merit but, if conducted without perspective, may be misleading because no evidence-based combination of antibody indicators consistently predicts future thrombotic events in SLE. Conventional therapeutic options are clear when there is a definitive history of a thrombotic event or typical pregnancy losses coupled with serologic evidence for APS. The more likely scenario encountered during routine screening in SLE is that one or more aCL, LAC, and anti-β2GPI antibodies will be detected. In the absence of convincing past history or clinical findings, this can create a therapeutic dilemma. The increasing evidence that the presence and persistence of anti-β2GPI is linked to future thrombosis [16,18,19] may provide the rationale for identifying patients at risk and pre-empting thrombosis (with the added benefit of slowing the emergence of premature atherosclerosis perhaps) with the use of low-dose aspirin and statin therapy.

The effect of APS on the clinical expression of SLE is now being realized [20,21]. Superimposed thrombotic complications like renal infarction and renal artery or vein thrombosis of APS can exacerbate the glomerulonephritis of SLE. Many of the earlier described central nervous system manifestations of SLE, especially seizures, strokes, and transverse myelitis, were most likely caused by endothelial perturbation and vaso-occlusive disease of APS and not SLE [22]. Pulmonary hypertension in patients who have SLE is also more likely secondary to APS [23].

A review in 2005 of 250 patients who had CAPS reported that almost 50% of them had SLE or lupus-like disease [24]. It is impossible to determine how many patients who have SLE/APS will develop CAPS because of the unavoidable case selection bias present in the literature. When CAPS does occur within the context of SLE, mortality appears to be higher [21].

The urgent clinical question of whether pre-emptive anticoagulation of SLE patients who have ominous aPL profiles will prevent APS needs to be resolved, but when definite APS is present in SLE, there is consensus that two different, but potentially complementary, treatment strategies be used. APS needs to be managed aggressively with anticoagulation while the immune complex pathogenesis of SLE is blunted with corticosteroid therapy combined with some form of B-cell suppression, usually cyclophosphamide (CTX) (Cytoxan), or mofetil mycophenolate (CellCept). The limitations of contemporary treatment regimens of SLE are many, not the least being lack of efficacy in many patients and toxicity in most. Although the fundamental problem in APS and SLE may be defective immunoregulation by T regulatory cells, the burgeoning literature on the efficacy of B-cell depletion with the CD20 monoclonal antibody rituximab (Rituxan) in SLE is encouraging because this strategy might simultaneously suppress the production of APS autoantibodies.

ANTIPHOSPHOLIPID ANTIBODY SYNDROME AND AUTOIMMUNE DISEASE: SJÖGREN'S SYNDROME

Primary Sjögren's syndrome (PSS), defined with revised criteria by the European Study Group in 2002 [25], is an autoimmune exocrinopathy with protean extraglandular organ manifestations and antibodies to Ro or La or both, and is characterized histologically by focal lymphocytic infiltration of exocrine glands. Many PSS patients have a plethora of autoantibodies, including those characteristic of APS. In the largest study to date, 13% of 281 patients who had PSS had some type of aPL [26]. Most of the aCL-positive patients had a wide range of IgM and IgG aCL and a significant number had LA. Unfortunately, anti-β2GPI antibodies were not measured in these patients. Almost three quarters of the aCL-positive PSS had extraglandular features and 6 of 36 progressed to definite or probable APS. Multiple other studies and case reports have tried to assess the significance of aPL in PSS. A unified clinical and serologic tabulation of these additional 98 PSS patients is nested within the report of Ramon-Casals and colleagues [26]. Anti-β2GPI antibody prevalence is not available in most of these studies. When anti-β2GPI antibodies have been determined in PSS, only 4% of 74 patients were positive in one study [27] and none of 80 patients were positive in another [28]. Overall, it is difficult to make a meaningful assessment of the true incidence of APS in PSS, but whatever the true frequency is, it is likely to be low. Longitudinal follow-up of aPL-positive patients who had PSS is insufficient to estimate how many aPL-positive ones evolve to APS. Secondary Sjögren's syndrome, a symptom complex similar to PSS but one occurring in the context of another autoimmune disease, usually SLE or RA, does not have any compelling differences from PSS in terms of autoantibody frequency. The presence of aPL more likely mirrors the frequency of aPL in the disease that the secondary Sjögren's syndrome is linked to, which appears to be the case in SLE [13].

ANTIPHOSPHOLIPID ANTIBODY SYNDROME AND AUTOIMMUNE DISEASE: RHEUMATOID ARTHRITIS

RA is a systemic inflammatory disease with a genetic predisposition and a clinical phenotype characterized by symmetric synovitis of large, medium, and small joints. Like many other autoimmune diseases, most RA patients have numerous autoantibodies that are generated by a loss of B-cell homeostasis. It is no surprise that aPL are found in RA [13,15,29–31], but the significance of aPL in RA remains to be determined. The frequency of aPL of any type ranges from 7% to 37%, and their presence does not correlate with a thrombotic state. When measured, anti-β2GPI antibodies were absent [30]. Two decades ago, a study of 243 patients revealed that 33% of those with RA were aCL positive and aCL-RA patients had a higher incidence of recurrent spontaneous abortions (70%) when compared with non–aCL RA patients (22%). The lack of matched control groups, the use of early-generation aCL testing, and other clinical variables make these correlations interesting observations only [28]. Another study found a strong correlation between the presence of rheumatoid nodules and aCL [31]. One suspects that this may not be a causal link but simply reflects the intense inflammation present in many RA patients before the widespread use of anti–tumor necrosis factor (TNF) α agents and low-dose corticosteroids. Neither APS nor CAPS is common in RA [32].

The contemporary use of TNFα antagonists has given rise to the interesting observation that 3 months or more of treatment with infliximab (Remicade), but not etanercept (Enbrel), is associated with an increased frequency of IgM and IgG aCL in RA [33]. Four patients in this study had thromboembolic events. Although these findings require confirmation, the emergence of aCL during TNFα antagonist treatment, coupled with the previously reported increase in antinuclear antibodies under similar circumstances [34], should alert the clinician to be wary of their confounding potential when they are used to treat RA.

For several reasons, interest may be renewed in aPL in RA. Reduced life expectancy and excess cardiovascular disease mortality occur in RA [35]. The cause is multifactorial, but the rapidly expanding awareness of interactions between aPL and lipoproteins [36] and aPL and endothelial perturbation [37] that can increase the potential for thrombosis suggest these autoantibodies may be more than just epiphenomena in RA. The presence of aPL may have importance outside the definitions of the APS syndrome [38]. They may be risk factors for premature atherosclerosis and increased cardiovascular mortality in RA and possibly other autoimmune diseases like SLE.

ANTIPHOSPHOLIPID ANTIBODY SYNDROME AND AUTOIMMUNE DISEASE: SYSTEMIC SCLEROSIS

Systemic sclerosis (SSc) or scleroderma is an autoimmune disease characterized clinically by ischemia-driven fibrosis of skin, gut, and lungs. The pathophysiology of SSc remains elusive, as does even a hint of an immunologic abnormality as its fundamental cause. For these reasons, attempts to identify subsets of scleroderma for the purposes of classification, prognosis, and therapy continue to be nettlesome issues [39]. Reports are limited on the occurrence of aPL in scleroderma. In a large cohort of patients who had connective tissue diseases, scleroderma patients had an aCL incidence of slightly less than 7%, a frequency no different than that of controls [13]. In a smaller study, SSc patients did have slightly elevated aCL levels when compared with controls but were markedly less positive than other patients who had SLE or Sjögren's syndrome [15]. A more recent study analyzed aCL in 68 patients who had SSc [40]. Almost one half had severe peripheral ischemia and 13 required amputation. Overall, the incidence of aCL was low and aCL frequency was no different between those who required surgery and those who did not. It would appear that neither APS nor CAPS is common in SSc.

The two clinical subsets of SSc are diffuse cutaneous scleroderma and limited cutaneous scleroderma (sometimes referred to as the CREST syndrome). Whether this clinical division is useful is being debated, but most rheumatologists, although agreeing that the two syndromes have significant overlap, believe that severe pulmonary hypertension is much more common in the limited form. A recent analysis of aCL and anti-β2GPI antibodies in 108 SSc patients sheds light on a possible etiologic factor that supports the clinical distinction between the diffuse and limited forms of scleroderma [23]. Although these results confirm those of older studies cited previously that aCL frequency is low, they provide new evidence that anti-β2GPI antibody prevalence is also low in SSc. The presence of aCL and pulmonary hypertension were significantly correlated, which supports the notion that aCL, causing chronic endothelial perturbation, can mediate more than just a thrombotic state. Additional circumstantial evidence of a possible link between aCL and endothelial damage can be found in two studies. In a small group of SLE patients who had aCL, 10 of 15 had Raynaud's phenomenon and 5 of 15 had livedo reticularis [14]. In another SLE cohort, aCL and nail fold capillary changes were correlated, prompting the investigators to suggest that aCL may damage vascular endothelium [15].

Almost 10 years ago, the prevalence of LAC, aCL, and anti-β2GPI antibodies was determined in 54 patients who had primary or secondary pulmonary hypertension, and there was a strong correlation of LAC, aCL, or anti-β2GPI antibody with thromboembolic pulmonary hypertension [41]. The link between procoagulant antibodies and in situ thrombosis in the pulmonary tree might seem self-evident, but it is now clear that some patients who have primary pulmonary hypertension have little or no in situ or embolic thrombosis. The possibility that LAC, aCL, and anti-β2GPI antibodies may increase local production of endothelin and cause pulmonary hypertension in the absence of actual thrombosis needs to be addressed. Until recently, the clinical relevance of detecting pulmonary hypertension and, to a lesser extent, Raynaud's phenomenon in diffuse and limited SSc was an academic exercise of sorts because limited therapeutic options were available. Now, with the availability of the phosphodiesterase inhibitor sildenafil and the dual endothelin antagonist bosentan, this is no longer true.

Patients who have so-called "idiopathic Raynaud's phenomenon" do not appear to have an increased frequency of aCL [42,43], and CAPS has no unique association with SSC.

ANTIPHOSPHOLIPID ANTIBODY SYNDROME AND AUTOIMMUNE DISEASE: SYSTEMIC VASCULITIS OTHER THAN SYSTEMIC LUPUS ERYTHEMATOSUS

APS is a vasculopathy, not a vasculitis. Vascular damage in APS is mediated by thrombosis and is not causally related to inflammation of the vascular wall [44]. In theory, the pathology of APS should be readily distinguishable from that of vasculitis but often this is difficult because secondary inflammation generated by the ischemic pathology of APS can mimic systemic vasculitis. The contention that a systemic vasculitis of any cause could predispose a patient to aCL-promoted thrombosis superimposed on the inflammation of a blood vessel has been difficult to prove. Inflammatory damage to the endothelium exposes phospholipid epitopes to aCL and it would seem logical that superimposed thrombosis might occur. The "which came first" question may never be answered, but the occurrence of thrombosis in a patient who has vasculitis from any cause should not be relegated automatically to an inflammatory cause but should prompt the clinician to consider superimposed APS. Case reports and retrospective group analyses of patients who had systemic vasculitis and APS are numerous, but all are unavoidably compromised by strong case selection bias. In a study of 80 patients who had giant cell arteritis (GCA) or polymyalgia rheumatica (PMR), 33% of patients who had GCA only, or GCA and PMR, had LAC, and no patient who had isolated PMR had the antibody [45]. No relationship could be found between ischemic symptoms and the presence of any kind of aPL. APS has been described in three patients who had GCA/PMR. The investigators made the important observation that clinical expression of either APS or GCA/PMR were not linked and treatment of one did not affect the other, suggesting that APS should be considered an independent disease [46]. Another study reported that 50% of patients who had acute temporal arteritis had IgG aCL. The aCL fell during treatment of the GCA with corticosteroids, which suggests that aCL emerge as an epiphenomenon or acute phase reactant during the inflammatory phase of GCA [47]. Low frequencies of aCL have been reported in a wide array of other systemic vasculitis, including anti neutrophil cytoplasmic antibodies positive renal vasculitis [13] and Wegener's granulomatosas [48]. The latter had no clinical manifestations of APS. Although APS has been described in patients who had polyarteritis nodosa or microscopic polyarteritis nodosa, no significant relationship between APS and either disease was found in several larger groups of patients [49-51]. The broad and heterogeneous spectrum of diseases associated with aPL but not APS prompted an editorial that made a very sensible case for regarding aPL as expected, unimportant, and probably not a group of tests that should be ordered routinely in systemic vascular disorders [44].

Tabulations of aCL in several other diseases of suspect autoimmune cause are available. Anecdotal reports describe the development of APS in one patient who had Behcet's disease, and CAPS in another [52,53]. Although 10 of 25 patients who had Behcet's disease had IgG aCL, there was no correlation with any of the numerous thrombotic complications in the patient group as a whole. Patients who have polymyositis have a frequency of aPL no higher than blood bank controls [13]. In two groups of patients who had either dermatomyositis or polymyositis, aPL was found to be higher than in controls but less than in SLE [14] in one group, and one of seven patients in the other had aPL [29].

In summary, the caveats that apply to the value of aPL detection in systemic vasculitis are also true for Behcet's disease and inflammatory muscle disease.

TREATMENT OF ANTIPHOSPHOLIPID ANTIBODY SYNDROME AND AUTOIMMUNE DISEASE

Before the treatment of APS in autoimmune diseases can be discussed, the complexities of making the diagnosis have to be addressed. The diagnosis of APS is based on the often difficult assessment of whether aPL, so frequently present in so many autoimmune diseases, are mediating clinical expression of thrombotic or pregnancy-related complications. Not all ischemic complications of appendages, the gut, and emboli in SLE, or the third trimester, are due to APS, and the clinician must maintain a perspective about the common occurrence of many types of aPL as epiphenomena in autoimmune diseases. The diagnosis of "secondary" APS is best made in the same context as the diagnosis of PAPS. The contemporary and conventional treatment of APS, whether primary or secondary, is anticoagulation. The treatment of secondary APS is done in parallel with, but independent of, treatment of the associated autoimmune disease. New approaches to the treatment of SLE, the disease most commonly associated with concomitant APS, may provide significant insight into better ways to treat APS.

The standard treatment of active SLE with significant renal or central nervous system involvement has been the use of CTX and corticosteroids. CTX inhibits proliferation of naïve and activated T cells by the direct induction of apoptosis [54]. The effect of CTX on B cells may involve direct apoptosis of B cells [55] and indirect loss of T helper cell signals. The pervasive opinion that self-reactive B-cell clones are depleted by CTX has never been proved in humans, but clinicians strongly believe that CTX therapy can reduce autoantibody titers to several self-antigens. When a small group of patients who had optic neuritis and SLE were treated with CTX, aCL in four patients decreased with treatment, and two of the four ultimately became aCL negative [56]. Despite all the studies documenting the prevalence of aPL in autoimmune diseases, not one has measured, as a primary outcome, the long-term effects of CTX on aCL in either PAPS or SLE/APS. Plasmapheresis, especially when used in conjunction with CTX [57], has been reported to be efficacious in CAPS and APS [58,59], but a systematic analysis has not been done of what effect CTX and plasmapheresis, when used for SLE, has on aPL or the emergence of APS.

The growing awareness that B-cell suppression may be effective in APS may be indirectly confirmed when the results of clinical trials using rituximab in SLE become available. The compelling logic for the use of the anti-CD20 monoclonal antibody in SLE should apply to an antibody-driven disease like APS. "Off-label" use of rituximab in SLE is already widespread and early clinical results are encouraging [60,61]. Many rheumatologists are devising protocols to exploit the synergistic effects of CTX therapy combined with rituximab. Over time, it may be shown that APS in CTX-rituximab–treated SLE is encountered much less frequently. Rituximab use in RA is also increasing rapidly and it will be interesting to see if aPL frequency decreases in these patients also.

Another novel pharmaceutic therapy is now being widely applied in patients who have SLE and RA that may influence the clinical expression of APS. The convincing epidemiologic evidence of premature atherosclerosis in SLE [62,63] and marked increase in cardiovascular mortality in RA make statin therapy an imperative in both diseases. Fluvastatin (Lescol) has been shown to inhibit in vitro anti-β2GPI antibody–mediated endothelial activation [64] and the expression of adhesion molecules on human monocytes [65], reduce the size of thrombi and the number of adherent leucocytes, and decrease serum levels of intercellular adhesion molecule in a murine APS model [66]. Whether the increasing use of statins in autoimmune diseases will indirectly reduce secondary APS is a tantalizing question that won't be answered for some time.

Autologous stem cell transplantation (ASCT) has been used in highly selected patients who have SLE. One patient who had SLE and APS went into remission for almost 2 years after ASCT [67]. Forty-six patients who have SLE have undergone ASCT [68]. Sixty-one percent of these patients also had features of APS. A significant portion of the patients who had aCL and LAC antibodies became seronegative after transplant. Most importantly, 18 of 22 patients who had been difficult to maintain appropriately anticoagulated were able to discontinue anticoagulation therapy within 4 months of transplantation. No cases of ASCT in patients who have PAPS have been reported. The encouraging results with novel approaches like rituximab and ASCT in refractory autoimmune diseases should encourage their consideration for use in PAPS and APS associated with autoimmune diseases.

SUMMARY

aPL are frequently encountered in SLE and, to a lesser extent, in other autoimmune diseases. In most instances, aPL represent an epiphenomenon of a dysregulated immune system but they can mediate APS, especially in SLE. Evidence is also mounting that aPL may not only be causally linked to pulmonary hypertension in SLE and scleroderma but also act as a cofactor in the accelerated atherosclerosis of autoimmune diseases.

References

[1] Asherson RA, Cervera R. Antiphospholipid antibodies and infections. Ann Rheum Dis 2002;62(5):388–93.
[2] Quemeneur T, Lambert M, Hachulla E, et al. Significance of persistent antiphospholipid antibodies in the elderly. J Rheumatol 2006;33(8):1559–62.
[3] Harris EN, Pierangeli SS. Primary, secondary, catastrophic antiphospholipid syndrome: is there a difference? Thromb Res 2004;114(5–6):357–61.
[4] Piette JC, Wechsler B, Frances C, et al. Systemic lupus erythematosus and the antiphospholipid syndrome: reflections about the relevance of ARA criteria. J Rheumatol 1992;19(12):1835–7.
[5] Asherson RA, Cervera R, Piette JC, et al. Catastrophic antiphospholipid syndrome: clues to the pathogenesis from a series of 80 patients. Medicine (Baltimore) 2001;80(6):355–77.
[6] Vianna JL, Khamashta MA, Ordi-Ros J, et al. Comparison of the primary and secondary antiphospholipid syndrome. A European multicenter study of 114 patients. Am J Med 1994;96(1):3–9.
[7] Alarcon-Segovia D, Perez-Vasquez ME, Villa AR, et al. Preliminary classification criteria for the antiphospholipid syndrome within systemic lupus erythematosus. Semin Arthritis Rheum 1992;21(5):275–86.
[8] Piette JC, Wechsler B, Frances C, et al. Exclusion criteria for primary antiphospholipid syndrome. J Rheumatol 1993;20(10):1802–4.
[9] Alarcon-Segovia D, Sanchez-Guerroro J. Primary antiphospholipid syndrome. J Rheumatol 1989;16(7):482–8.
[10] Grossman JM. Primary versus secondary antiphospholipid syndrome: is this lupus or not? Curr Rheumatol Rep 2004;6(6):445–50.
[11] Lockshin MD, Sammaritano LR, Schwartzman S. Validation of the Sapporo criteria for antiphospholipid syndrome. Arthritis Rheum 2000;43(2):440–3.
[12] Cervera R, Piette JC, Font J, et al. Antiphospholipid syndrome: clinical and immunologic manifestations and patterns of disease expression in a cohort of 1000 patients. Arthritis Rheum 2002;46(4):1019–27.
[13] Merkel PA, Chang Y, Pierangeli SS, et al. The prevalence and clinical associations of anticardiolipin antibodies in a large inception cohort of patients with connective tissue diseases. Am J Med 1996;101(6):576–83.
[14] Buchanan RR, Wardlaw JR, Riglar AG, et al. Antiphospholipid antibodies in the connective tissue diseases: their relation to the antiphospholipid syndrome and forme fruste disease. J Rheumatol 1989;16(6):757–61.
[15] Bongard O, Boumaneaux H, Miescher PA, et al. Association of anticardiolipin antibodies and abnormal nailfold capillaroscopy in patients with systemic lupus erythematosus. Lupus 1995;4(2):142–4.
[16] Danowski A, Kickler TS, Petri M. Anti-β2-glycoprotein I: prevalence, clinical correlations, and importance of persistent positivity in patients with antiphospholipid syndrome and systemic lupus erythematosus. J Rheumatol 2006;33(9):1775–9.
[17] McMahon MA, Keogan M, O'Connell P, et al. The prevalence of antiphospholipid antibody syndrome among systemic lupus erythematosus patients. Ir Med J 2006;100(9):296–8.
[18] Yasuda S, Atsumi T, Iako M, et al. β2-glycoprotein I, anti-β2-glycoprotein I, and fibrinolysis. Thromb Res 2004;114(5–6):461–5.
[19] Miyakis S, Lockshin MD, Atsumi T, et al. International consensus statement on an update of the classification criteria for definite antiphospholipid syndrome (APS). J Thromb Haemost 2006;4(2):295–306.
[20] Laskin CA, Clark CA, Spitzer KA. Antiphospholipid syndrome in systemic lupus erythematosus: is the whole greater than the sum of its parts? Rheum Clin Dis North Am 2005;31(2):255–72.

[21] Bucciarelli S, Espinosa G, Cervera R, et al. Mortality in the catastrophic antiphospholipid syndrome: causes of death and prognostic factors in a series of 250 patients. Arthritis Rheum 2006;54(8):2568–76.
[22] Lavalle C, Pizarro S, Drenkard C, et al. Transverse myelitis: a manifestation of systemic lupus erythematosus strongly associated with antiphospholipid antibodies. J Rheumatol 1990;17(1):34–7.
[23] Assous N, Allanore Y, Batteux F, et al. Prevalence of antiphospholipid antibodies in systemic sclerosis and association with primitive pulmonary arterial hypertension and endothelial injury. Clin Exp Rheumatol 2005;23(2):199–204.
[24] Asherson RA. Multiorgan failure and antiphospholipid antibodies: the catastrophic antiphospholipid (Asherson's) syndrome. Immunobiology 2005;210(10):727–33.
[25] Vitali C, Bombardieri S, Jonsson R, et al. Classification criteria for Sjögren syndrome: a revised version of the European criteria proposed by the American-European Consensus Group. Ann Rheum Dis 2002;61(6):554–8.
[26] Ramos-Casals M, Nardi N, Brito-Zeron P, et al. Atypical autoantibodies in patients with primary Sjogren syndrome: clinical characteristics and follow-up of 82 cases. Semin Arthritis Rheum 2006;35(5):312–21.
[27] Fauchais AL, Lambert M, Launay D, et al. Antiphospholipid antibodies in primary Sjogren's syndrome: prevalence and clinical significance in a series of 74 patients. Lupus 2004;13(4):245–8.
[28] Cervera R, Garcia-Carrasco M, Font J, et al. Antiphospholipid antibodies in primary Sjogren's syndrome: prevalence and clinical significance in a series of 80 patients. Clin Exp Rheumatol 1997;15(4):361–5.
[29] Fort JG, Cowchock S, Abruzzo JL, et al. Anticardiolipin antibodies in patients with rheumatic diseases. Arthritis Rheum 1987;30(7):752–60.
[30] Vittecoq O, Jouen-Beades F, Krzanowska K, et al. Prospective evaluation of the frequency and clinical significance of antineutrophil cytoplasmic and anticardiolipin antibodies in community cases of patients with rheumatoid arthritis. Rheumatology 2000;39(5):481–9.
[31] Wolf P, Gretler J, Aglas F, et al. Anticardiolipin antibodies in rheumatoid arthritis: their relation to rheumatoid nodules and cutaneous vascular manifestations. Br J Dermatol 1994;131(1):48–51.
[32] Asherson RA, Cervera R, Piette JC, et al. Catastrophic antiphospholipid syndrome: clinical and laboratory features of 50 patients. Medicine (Baltimore) 1998;77(3):195–207.
[33] Jonsdottir T, Forslid J, van Vollenhoven A, et al. Treatment with tumour necrosis factor alpha antagonists in patients with rheumatoid arthritis induces anticardiolipin antibodies. Ann Rheum Dis 2004;63(9):1075–8.
[34] De Rycke L, Baeten D, Kruithof E, et al. The effect of TNF alpha blockade on the antinuclear antibody profile in patients with chronic arthritis: biological and clinical implications. Lupus 2005;14(12):931–7.
[35] Goodson N, Marks J, Lunt M, et al. Cardiovascular admissions and mortality in an inception cohort of patients with rheumatoid arthritis with onset in the 1980s and 1990s. Ann Rheum Dis 2005;64(11):1595–601.
[36] Seriolo B, Accardo S, Fasciolo D, et al. Lipoproteins, anticardiolipin antibodies and thrombotic events in rheumatoid arthritis. Clin Exp Rheumatol 1996;14(6):593–9.
[37] Wallberg-Jonsson S, Cvetkovic JT, Sundqvist KG, et al. Activation of the immune system and inflammatory activity in relation to markers of atherothrombotic disease and atherosclerosis in rheumatoid arthritis. J Rheumatol 2002;29(5):875–82.
[38] Shoenfeld Y, Gerli R, Doria A, et al. Accelerated atherosclerosis in autoimmune rheumatic diseases. Ann N Y Acad Sci 2005;1122(21):3337–47, 1051.
[39] Wollheim F. Classification of systemic sclerosis. Visions and reality. Rheumatology 2005;44(10):1212–6.

[40] Herrick AL, Heaney M, Hollis S, et al. Anticardiolipin, anticentromere and anti-Scl-70 antibodies in patients with systemic sclerosis and severe digital ischaemia. Ann Rheum Dis 1995;53(8):540–2.
[41] Martinuzzo ME, Pombo G, Forastiero RR. Lupus anticoagulant, high levels of cardiolipin, and anti-beta2- glycoprotein I antibodies are associated with chronic thromboembolic pulmonary hypertension. J Rheumatol 1998;25(7):1313–9.
[42] Manoussakis MN, Gharavi AE, Drosos AA, et al. Anticardiolipin antibodies in unselected autoimmune rheumatic disease patients. Clin Immunol Immunopathol 1987;44(3):297–307.
[43] Asherson RA, Mayou SC, Merry P, et al. The spectrum of livedo reticularis and anticardiolipin antibodies. Br J Dermatol 1989;120(2):215–21.
[44] Cuchacovich R, Espinoza LR. Is antiphospholipid antibody determination clinically relevant to the vasculitides? Semin Arthritis Rheum 2001;31(1):1–3.
[45] Espinosa G, Tassies D, Font J, et al. Antiphospholipid antibodies and thrombophilic factors in giant cell arteritis. Semin Arthritis Rheum 2001;31(1):12–20.
[46] Ruffatti A, Montecucco C, Volante D, et al. Antiphospholipid antibody syndrome and polymyalgia rheumatica/giant cell arteritis. Rheumatol 2000;39(5):565–7.
[47] McHugh NJ, James IE, Plant GT. Anticardiolipin and antineutrophil antibodies in giant cell arteritis. J Rheumatol 1990;17(7):916–22.
[48] Meyer MF, Schnabel A, Schatz H, et al. Lack of association between antiphospholipid antibodies and thrombocytopenia in patients with Wegener's granulomatosis. Semin Arthritis Rheum 2001;31(1):4–11.
[49] Handa R, Aggarwal P, Biswas A, et al. Microscopic polyangiitis associated with antiphospholipid syndrome. Rheumatology 1999;38(5):478–9.
[50] Norden DK, Ostrov BE, Shafritz AB, et al. Vasculitis associated with antiphospholipid syndrome. Semin Arthritis Rheum 1995;24(4):273–81.
[51] Dasgupta B, Almond MK, Tanqueray A. Polyarteritis nodosa and the antiphospholipid syndrome. Br J Rheumatol 1997;36(11):1210–2.
[52] Famularo G, Antonelli S, Barracchini A, et al. Catastrophic antiphospholipid syndrome in a patient with Behcet's disease. Scand J Rheumatol 2002;31(2):100–2.
[53] Mader R, Ziv M, Adawi M, et al. Thrombophilic factors and their relation to thromboembolic and other clinical manifestations in Behcet's disease. J Rheumatol 1999;26(11):2404–8.
[54] Strauss G, Osen W, Debatin K-M. Induction of apoptosis and modulation of activation and effector function in T cells by immunosuppressive drugs. Clin Exp Immunol 2002;128(2):255–66.
[55] Hemendinger RA, Bloom SE. Selective mitomycin C and cyclophosphamide induction of apoptosis in differentiating B lymphocytes compared to T lymphocytes in vivo. Immunopharmacology 1996;35(1):71–82.
[56] Galindo-Rodriguez G, Avina-Subieta A, Pizarro S, et al. Cyclophosphamide pulse therapy in optic neuritis due to systemic lupus erythematosus: an open trial. Am J Med 1999;106(1):65–9.
[57] Koschmieder S, Miesbach W, Fauth F, et al. Combined plasmapheresis and immunosuppression as rescue treatment of a patient with catastrophic antiphospholipid syndrome occurring despite anticoagulation: a case report. Blood Coagul Fibrinolysis 2003;14(4):395–9.
[58] Lacueva J, Enriquez R, Cabezuelo JB, et al. Acute renal failure as first clinical manifestation of the primary antiphospholipid syndrome. Nephron 1993;64(3):479–80.
[59] Yagi K, Kawano M, Haraki T, et al. Long-term efficacy of immunoadsorbent plasmapheresis in a patient with Budd-Chiari syndrome due to antiphospholipid syndrome: case report with nine-year follow up. Lupus 2004;13(2):135–8.
[60] Marks SD, Patey S, Brogan PA, et al. B lymphocyte depletion therapy in children with refractory systemic lupus erythematosus. Arthritis Rheum 2005;52(10):3168–74, B.

[61] Smith KG, Jones RB, Burns SM, et al. Long-term comparison of rituximab treatment for refractory systemic lupus erythematosus and vasculitis: remission, relapse and retreatment. Arthritis Rheum 2006;54(9):2970–82, B.
[62] Vlachoyiannopoulos PG, Kanellopoulos PG, Ioannidis PA, et al. Atherosclerosis in premenopausal women with antiphospholipid syndrome and systemic lupus erythematosus: a controlled study. Rheumatology 2003;42(5):645–51.
[63] Manzi S, Selzer F, Sutton-Tyrrell K. Prevalence and risk factors of carotid plaque in women with systemic lupus erythematosus. Arthritis Rheum 1999;42(1):51–60.
[64] Meroni PL, Raschi E, Testoni C, et al. Statins prevent endothelial cell activation induced by antiphospholipid (anti-β2-glycoprotein I) antibodies: effect on the proadhesive and proinflammatory phenotype. Arthritis Rheum 2001;44(12):2870–8.
[65] Niwa S, Totsuka T, Hayashi S. Inhibitory effect of fluvastatin, an HMG-CoA reductase inhibitor on the expression of adhesion molecules on human monocyte cell line. Int J Immunopharmacol 1996;18(11):669–75.
[66] Ferrara DE, Liu X, Espinola RG, et al. Inhibition of the thrombogenic and inflammatory properties of antiphospholipid antibodies by fluvastatin in an in vivo animal model. Arthritis Rheum 2003;48(11):3272–9.
[67] Hashimoto N, Iwasaki T, Sekiguchi M, et al. Autologous hematopoietic stem cell transplantation for refractory antiphospholipid syndrome causing myocardial necrosis. Bone Marrow Transplant 2004;33(8):863–6, B.
[68] Statkute L, Traynor A, Oyama Y, et al. Antiphospholipid syndrome in patients with systemic lupus erythematosus treated by autologous hematopoietic stem cell transplantation. Blood 2005;106(8):2700–9.

Cutaneous Manifestations of Antiphospholipid Antibody Syndrome

Sari Weinstein, MD[a], Warren Piette, MD[a,b],*

[a]Division of Dermatology, John H. Stroger, Jr. Hospital of Cook County, 1900 West Polk Street, Room 519, Chicago, IL 60612, USA
[b]Department of Dermatology, Rush University Medical Center, Annex Building, Suite 220, 707 S. Wood, Chicago, IL 60612, USA

Although no skin finding is pathognomonic for antiphospholipid antibody syndrome (APS), many cutaneous findings can be helpful in suggesting this diagnostic possibility. The cutaneous syndromes that should prompt consideration of APS are the focus of this article.

LIVEDO RETICULARIS AND RACEMOSA

Livedo reticularis is the most frequently associated cutaneous manifestation in patients who have APS, observed as the presenting sign in up to 40% of patients and seen in up to 70% of patients who have systemic lupus erythematosus (SLE) and APS [1]. In patients who have SLE, the finding of moderate-to-extensive livedo reticularis probably warrants testing for antiphospholipid antibodies (aPLs). In a recent consensus statement on the updated classification criteria for APS, Miyakis and colleagues [2] defined livedo reticularis as the persistent, not reversible with rewarming, violaceous, red or blue, reticular or mottled pattern of the skin of the trunk, arms, or legs. It may consist of regular, unbroken circles (regular livedo reticularis), or irregular, broken circles (livedo racemosa). The livedo patterns were further classified, depending on the width of branching pattern (greater or less than 10 mm), into fine and large livedo reticularis and fine and large livedo racemosa. Although the terms are frequently used interchangeably, compared with livedo reticularis, livedo racemosa is a coarser and more irregular pattern, is more often irregularly distributed, and may be more generalized (Fig. 1). Some investigators believe the racemosa variant to be a major clinical feature of APS, strongly associated with the arterial subset of APS, which includes cerebrovascular events, arterial

*Corresponding author. Division of Dermatology, John H. Stroger, Jr. Hospital of Cook County, 1900 West Polk Street, Room 519, Chicago, IL 60612. E-mail address: wpiette@cchil.org (W. Piette).

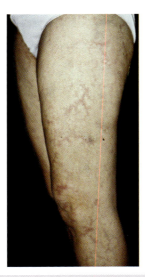

Fig. 1. Livedo. Sneddon's syndrome with widespread livedo. Although focal areas have a mostly regular reticulate pattern (eg, knee), most areas have a less regular, coarse pattern of racemosa.

thrombosis, systemic hypertension, heart valve abnormalities, Raynaud's phenomenon, and pregnancy morbidity, and consider it an independent, additive, thrombotic risk factor [1,3]. Livedo reticularis has been observed less frequently in those who have only venous thrombosis.

An impairment of blood flow and lowered oxygen tension at the periphery of skin segments is responsible for the mottling observed clinically. The cutaneous blood supply is arranged in inverted cones supplied by a central arteriole arising perpendicularly from vessels in the fascia. This arteriole is responsible for the blood supply to a 1- to 4-cm–diameter zone on the skin surface. The netlike pattern results from cyanotic discoloration at the junctions between cones, where deoxygenated blood accumulates. The ring size of the reticulate pattern depends on the body site and is usually smallest on the palms and largest on the trunk or thighs.

The pathophysiology of livedo is not well characterized, but the relationship with arterial thrombosis suggests a possible role for the endothelial cell. The vasoconstriction of livedo racemosa may be induced by an interaction of an aPL with the endothelial cell or other cellular element of vessels, altering their function [1,4]. Many autoantibodies associated with APS are directed against phospholipid-protein complexes expressed on, or bound to, the surface of endothelial cells. When bound, these cells may become prothrombotic, leading to the production of procoagulant substances such as tissue factor, plasminogen activator inhibitor 1, and endothelin 1; the increased expression of these procoagulants may be responsible, in part, for the hypercoagulability and thromboses observed in APS.

Unfortunately, livedo reticularis is a nonspecific cutaneous finding. In neonates, generalized livedo reticularis is an expected finding, termed cutis marmorata. Physiologic livedo reticularis in adults is common, triggered by cold and reversed by warming. Associations of nonphysiologic livedo reticularis with systemic diseases or medications are many; one recent review cited just short of 100 conditions [5].

IDIOPATHIC LIVEDO RETICULARIS WITH CEREBROVASCULAR ACCIDENTS (SNEDDON'S SYNDROME)

In 1965, Sneddon reported the association of livedo reticularis or racemosa with cerebrovascular accidents [6]. Sneddon's syndrome is a rare, but potentially severe, condition typically affecting young or middle-aged women, with the first cerebrovascular accident typically occurring before 45 years of age. Livedo of either type, typically on the trunk and buttocks but also on the extremities and face, may precede the onset of stroke by years. Although the relationship between APS and Sneddon's syndrome is not clear, the prevalence of aPLs in Sneddon's syndrome has ranged from 0% to 85%, and most authorities suggest that 40% to 50% of patients who have Sneddon's are antibody positive [1].

Skin biopsies are often nondiagnostic in Sneddon's syndrome. Multiple deep punch biopsies from the center and the violaceous areas are required to increase sensitivity. According to Zelger and colleagues [4], small-to-medium–sized arteries at the dermal-subcutis boundary are involved in a stage-specific pattern. Initial lesions are characterized by the attachment of lymphohistiocytic cells and the detachment of endothelial cells (endotheliitis). Early-phase lesions display partial or complete occlusion of vascular lumens by a plug of lymphohistiocytic cells and fibrin. Intermediate-phase lesions show replacement of plug by proliferating subendothelial cells and dilated capillaries in the adventitia of the occluded vessel. Late-phase lesions show fibrosis and shrinkage of vessels [1]. True vasculitis is not a feature.

Sneddon's syndrome may have two distinct causes, one aPL related with preferential arteriolar involvement, the other a primary non–aPL-related small artery disease primarily affecting the brain and skin vessels [7].

No treatment has consistently been effective for livedo. In patients who have Sneddon's or APS, chronic anticoagulation may be warranted, even though the livedo may worsen on anticoagulant or antiplatelet therapy. In light of the higher association of arterial occlusion in patients who have livedo racemosa, patients should reduce other risk factors, including smoking and use of estrogen-containing oral contraceptives. Low-dose aspirin is frequently prescribed, although its efficacy is unproven [8]. Further study is needed on the potential benefit of clopidogrel, statins, and angiotensin-converting enzyme inhibitors.

ATROPHIE BLANCHE AND LIVEDOID VASCULOPATHY

Atrophie blanche is a term that has been used for several different conditions, leading to some confusion in the literature. Originally described as atrophie blanche en plaque by Milian in 1929, synonyms for this disease include livedo reticularis with summer ulcerations; segmental hyalinizing vasculitis; livedo vasculitis; livedoid vasculitis; hypersensitivity-type vasculitis; and painful purpuric ulcers with reticular pattern of the lower extremities (PURPLE) [9–11]. The disease is often chronic, with seasonal exacerbations.

Idiopathic atrophie blanche (or white atrophy) is most often seen in young to middle-aged women, typically presenting as disproportionately painful lesions around the malleoli that rapidly progress to punched-out ulcers roughly 3 to 8 mm in diameter (Fig. 2). Within a few days to weeks, the ulcer margin is surrounded by punctate telangiectasias. These ulcers can be persistent but usually heal eventually with a porcelain white scar surrounded by telangiectasias. When presenting in this location, in women, and in this age group, without any systemic findings, aPLs are seldom associated.

The term atrophie blanche has also been applied to the white macules, typically less than 1 cm in diameter, that may be seen on the legs of individuals who have prominent varicosities. Because these lesions typically develop without an antecedent ulcer or pain, do not have surrounding telangiectasias, and do not appear to be associated with any coagulopathy, the term pseudo–atrophie blanche might be better applied to these sorts of lesions. Livedoid vasculopathy is a more extensive variant of atrophie blanche in which individual punctuate ulcers link with reticulate erythema or purpura to form areas several cm in diameter. The epidemiology for idiopathic and secondary forms is identical to that of atrophie blanche.

The histopathology of atrophie blanche and livedoid vasculopathy shows fibrin deposition within the walls and lumens of affected superficial dermal vessels, often with hyalinization of vessel walls. Thrombus within the lumen and red cell extravasation may be present, but the absence of a perivascular infiltrate or leukocytoclasia argues against a true vasculitis. Late-stage lesions may show epidermal atrophy with thickened hyalinized vessels [9].

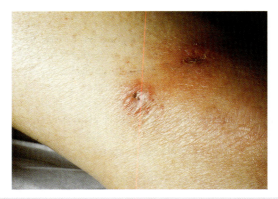

Fig. 2. Atrophie blanche. Two lesions of atrophie blanche near the ankle. One has healed with white scar. Expected telangiectasias are not prominent in this patient.

The pathogenesis of livedoid vasculopathy and atrophie blanche is unknown but it is believed to involve some altered local or systemic control of coagulation [11]. Many studies support a vaso-occlusive pathogenesis, and elevated fibrinopeptide A levels, defective release of vascular plasminogen activator, and decreased thrombomodulin expression have been described [9]. Livedoid vasculopathy is observed in patients who have procoagulant proclivities, including factor V Leiden, hyperhomocysteinemia, altered fibrinolysis or platelet activation, and aPLs [11]. However, control patients are seldom included in these reports, so it is unclear whether multiple screenings simply increase the discovery of incidental abnormalities.

Treatment of idiopathic atrophie blanche usually begins with aspirin, other antiplatelet agents, or pentoxifylline (Trental). When these fail, treatment is difficult. Minimally androgenic anabolic steroids have occasionally been helpful. A regimen of phenformin and anabolic steroid has been used successfully, but metformin does not appear to have similar efficacy [12].

Atrophie blanche–like lesions are seen in lupus patients, typically in association with aPLs, so the presence of such lesions should always prompt an APS workup in these patients. They are also seen in nonlupus patients who have APS, so a workup should be considered in patients with typical atrophie blanche lesions who are older, male, or who have lesions in sites other than perimalleolar areas.

No consensus exists regarding the treatment of livedoid vasculopathy in the setting of APS, although treatment to prevent further thromboses is probably indicated. Anecdotal success has been reported with antiplatelet, anticoagulant, and fibrinolytic therapies, including tissue plasminogen activator [11,13]. Hydroxychloroquine appears to be helpful in some lupus patients who have atrophie blanche–type lesions (personal observation), and appeared to reduce the risk of thrombosis in a large lupus cohort [14].

MALIGNANT ATROPHIC PAPULOSIS (DEGOS' DISEASE)

Malignant atrophic papulosis, also known as Degos' disease, is a rare, vaso-occlusive disorder that predominately affects the skin initially, followed by the gastrointestinal tract and central nervous system. Affected men outnumber women three to one [15]. Visceral lesions may result in fatal bowel and cerebral infarctions. Some cases of only cutaneous involvement have been reported. Mucous membranes, particularly the conjunctiva, may be involved. Skin lesions begin as crops of 2- to 5-mm pale rose or yellowish-gray firm papules on the trunk and extremities that evolve over 2 to 4 weeks with the development of a central depression and ultimately a porcelain white scar, often with a rim of telangiectasias. The end-stage appearance is very similar to that of atrophie blanche. It is unclear from the literature how many patients with "benign" Degos' disease, or skin-limited disease have been tested for aPLs. Degos-like lesions can be a cutaneous presentation of APS [16]. Patients who have such lesions, especially without visceral or central nervous system disease, should probably be investigated for the presence of aPLs.

Histologically, the classic description is that of an inverted, wedge-shaped zone of dermal infarction whose base is in contact with the overlying epidermis and apex is adjacent to a thrombosed vessel in the deep dermis. However, the classic histopathology occurs in only a minority of biopsies, and additional features must be sought, such as lymphocytic vasculitis; dermal mucin deposition; perineural and intraneural lymphocytic infiltrates; perivascular and periadnexal lymphocytic infiltrates; atrophy and compact hyperkeratosis of the epidermis; dermal–epidermal interface changes, including vacuolar change and necrotic basal keratinocytes; and sclerosing panniculitis [17]. The dermis may show frank necrosis or edema, mucin deposition, and slight sclerosis [18].

The pathogenesis of Degos' disease is unclear; the three main theories are viral, autoimmune, and coagulation abnormality. Raised circulating levels of fibrinogen and cryoprofibrin, and increased platelet aggregation and adhesiveness, have been reported in patients with Degos' disease [15].

Case reports have shown variable responses to antiplatelet therapy (aspirin, dipyridamole, and heparin), systemic corticosteroids, cyclophosphamide, azathioprine, phenformin, and ethylestrenol, and thus, no definitive treatment exists [15]. It is unknown how often responsive cases are associated with aPLs.

CATASTROPHIC ANTIPHOSPHOLIPID SYNDROME

The catastrophic APS, also known as CAPS, is a quickly progressing, often lethal manifestation first defined in 1992; in 2003, it also became known as Asherson's syndrome. Most often encountered in patients who have APS without lupus (49.9%), but also commonly in patients who have SLE and "lupus-like disease" (45%), this condition is characterized by rapid onset, resulting in multiple organ dysfunction; small-vessel occlusive disease with thrombotic microangiopathy; fulminant tissue necrosis, particularly in the gastrointestinal tract; and evidence of the systemic inflammatory response syndrome. Disseminated intravascular coagulation is also present in many patients [19].

The clinical appearance is similar to that of purpura fulminans, with widespread hemorrhagic infarction of the skin and intravascular thrombosis. Retiform (branching, stellate) purpura or eschar, usually noninflammatory, is a typical cutaneous lesion of most cutaneous microvascular occlusion syndromes, and APS and CAPS are no exception (Fig. 3) [11,18,20]. The organs involved clinically are renal (70%), pulmonary (66%), brain (60%), heart (52%), and skin (47%). It may arise in patients already diagnosed with APS and undergoing treatment, or in patients never before identified. Triggers identified in nearly two thirds of patients include infections; trauma, including minor surgical procedures such as biopsies; obstetric-related complications; anticoagulation withdrawal; neoplasia; and drugs. Treatment includes intravenous gamma globulins, plasma exchanges, high-dose intravenous steroids, fibrinolytic agents, and fresh-frozen plasma. The use of rituximab in patients with severe thrombocytopenia has also been successful [19]. A review of 250 patients with CAPS has been organized by the Europhospholipid Group and is available at http://www.med.ub.es/mimmun/forum/caps.htm [21]. Some

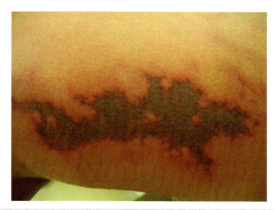

Fig. 3. Retiform. Purpura lesion is mostly nonblanchable. The retiform branching pattern is typical of most cutaneous microvascular occlusive lesions.

cases of CAPS have been called symmetric peripheral gangrene, but this acral presentation is not unique to APS.

PAPULAR AND PLAQUE OCCLUSIVE LESIONS

Cutaneous necrosis is another common manifestation of APS and may be second only to livedo reticularis in frequency. In the Cervera and colleagues [22] series, necrotic skin ulcerations were observed in 5.5% of patients who had APS and were the presenting sign in close to 4%. Lesions in Fig. 3 are typical of this presentation. The most commonly involved sites are the upper and lower extremities and helices of ears, cheeks, trunk, and forehead [22]; lesions may be widespread. The onset is often acute, with painful purpura [3]. Retiform (branching, stellate) lesions are typical of this presentation [11,18,20]. Occasionally, some lesions may have peripheral erythema, and necrotic bullae may form in affected areas. Pathology reveals diffuse, noninflammatory thrombosis of dermal vessels without evidence of vasculitis [3,23]. Many investigators regard widespread necrosis as a major thrombotic event, warranting long-term anticoagulation with an international normalized ratio higher than three, with or without low-dose aspirin [23].

Cutaneous digital gangrene, with preceding ischemic symptoms, has also been observed in up to 7.5% of patients with APS, and requires full anticoagulation [16,22].

Subungual splinter hemorrhages have been reported, appearing concurrently with thrombotic events or lupus flares [16].

Many nonspecific skin lesions, including red macules, purpura, small red or cyanotic lesions on the hands and feet, localized necrosis, ecchymoses, and painful skin nodules are also observed; these may be readily mischaracterized clinically as "vasculitis" if a biopsy is not taken. These pseudovasculitis lesions were the presenting manifestations in 2.6% of subjects in a European cohort

[22]. For such isolated lesions, combination therapy with low-dose aspirin and dipyridamole has been reported to be effective in some cases, but anticoagulation is usually prescribed.

ANETODERMA

Primary anetoderma is a rare skin disease of unknown cause characterized by loss of elastic fibers in the skin. Also known as macular atrophy, it was first described by Jadassohn in 1892. Lesions typically appear on the upper trunk and proximal extremities, presenting as multiple round, well-circumscribed, finely wrinkled patches or papules of slack skin that appear sunken, atrophied, or flaccid and demonstrate inward herniation or loss of substance on palpation (Figs. 4 and 5). Histopathologic examination of lesions should confirm decreased-to-absent elastic fibers in the upper and middle dermis, but requires special stains, usually Verhoeff-van Gieson elastin stain. Elastophagocytosis may be present [24].

Anetoderma is an uncommon syndrome that is most often idiopathic (primary) or develops at sites of inflammation (secondary) from many dermatoses, most commonly acne and varicella [25]. For more than 20 years, anetoderma has been reported in patients with connective tissue disease, especially SLE. The association of anetoderma and APS was first described by Hodak and colleagues [26] and Disdier and colleagues [27] in the early 1990s; since then, nearly two dozen reports have described patients presenting with both conditions. Other systemic associations include multiple autoimmune diseases (SLE; discoid lupus; lupus profundus; systemic sclerosis; vitiligo; alopecia

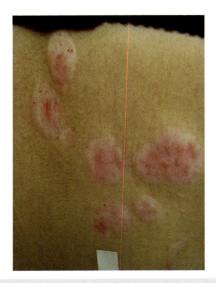

Fig. 4. Anetoderma. Clustered lesions on midback. Lesions are typically pale, soft, and flaccid.

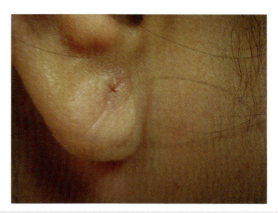

Fig. 5. Anetoderma. Close-up anetoderma on ear lobe.

areata; primary hypothyroidism with antithyroid antibodies; multiple sclerosis; and primary Addison's disease) and infections (HIV, syphilis, tuberculosis, and Lyme disease) [25]. It is still unclear what role, if any, aPLs play in the pathogenesis of anetoderma. However, several investigators suggest that the presence of anetoderma may warrant a workup for autoimmune disease and, in particular, APS [28].

Its association with so many immunologic abnormalities suggests an immunologic mechanism for the elastolysis observed. One hypothesis is an increased release or activation of elastase by inflammatory cells; others suggest loss of elastic fibers due to phagocytosis by macrophages, or reduced synthesis of elastic fibers; another theory suggests that microthrombosis in dermal vessels leads to local ischemia followed by degeneration of elastic fibers [29,30]. Some investigators propose a possible common epitope between elastic fibers and phospholipids (possibly beta-2GP1) as an explanation for an autoimmune-mediated process [31]. Recently, an abnormal balance between tissue metalloproteinases and tissue inhibitors has been demonstrated in anetodermic skin; the investigators suggest hypoxia reoxygenation in the skin may trigger a local imbalance of metalloproteinases and their inhibitors, leading to elastic tissue destruction.

Treatment of anetoderma is difficult. Multiple modalities have been attempted without consistent success, including topical and intralesional corticosteroids, penicillin G sodium, dapsone, colchicine, phenytoin, salicylates, hydroxychloroquine, and vitamin E [24,30].

References

[1] Uthman I, Khamashta M. Livedo racemosa: a striking dermatological sign for the antiphospholipid syndrome. J Rheumatol 2006;33(12):2379–82.

[2] Miyakis S, Lockshin M, Atsumi T, et al. International consensus statement on an update of the classification criteria for definite antiphospholipid syndrome (APS). J Thromb Haemost 2005;4:295–306.

[3] Frances C, Niang S, Laffitte E, et al. Dermatologic manifestations of the antiphospholipid syndrome. Arthritis Rheum 2005;52:1785–90.
[4] Zelger B, Sepp N, Stockhammer G, et al. Sneddon's syndrome: long-term follow-up of 21 patients. Arch Dermatol 1993;129:437–47.
[5] Gibbs M, English J, Zirwas M. Livedo reticularis: an update. J Am Acad Dermatol 2005;52(6):1009–19.
[6] Sneddon I. Cerebro-vascular lesions and livedo reticularis. Br J Dermatol 1965;77:180–5.
[7] Frances C, Piette JC. The mystery of Sneddon syndrome: relationship with antiphospholipid syndrome and systemic lupus erythematosus. J Autoimmun 2000;15(2):139–43.
[8] Erkan D, Harrison MJ, Levy R, et al. Aspirin for primary thrombosis prevention in the antiphospholipid syndrome: a randomized, double-blind, placebo-controlled trial in asymptomatic antiphospholipid antibody-positive individuals. Arthritis Rheum 2007;56(7):2383–91.
[9] Acland KM, Darvay A, Wakelin SH, et al. Livedoid vasculitis: a manifestation of the antiphospholipid syndrome? Br J Dermatol 1999;140(1):131–5.
[10] Hairston B, Davis M, Pittelkow M, et al. Livedoid vasculopathy: further evidence for procoagulant pathogenesis. Arch Dermatol 2006;142:1413–8.
[11] Piette W. Cutaneous manifestations of microvascular occlusion syndromes. In: Bolognia J, Jorrizo J, Rapini R, editors. Dermatology. 1st edition. London: Mosby; 2003. p. 2003.
[12] Shornick J, Nicholes B, Bergstresser P, et al. Idiopathic atrophie blanche. J Am Acad Dermatol 1983;8(6):792–8.
[13] Klein K, Pittelkow M. Tissue plasminogen activator for treatment of livedoid vasculitis. Mayo Clin Proc 1992;67:923–33.
[14] Petri M. Hydroxychloroquine use in the Baltimore Lupus Cohort: effects on lipids, glucose and thrombosis. Lupus 1996;5(Suppl 1):S16–22.
[15] Katz S, Mudd L, Roenigk H. Malignant atrophic papulosis (Degos' disease) involving three generations of a family. J Am Acad Dermatol 1997;37:480–4.
[16] Gibson G, Su W, Pittelkow M. Antiphospholipid syndrome and the skin. J Am Acad Dermatol 1997;36:970–82.
[17] Harvell J, Williford P, White W. Benign cutaneous Degos' disease: a case report with emphasis on histopathology as papules chronologically evolve. Am J Dermatopathol 2001;23(2):116–23.
[18] Robson K, Piette W. The presentation and differential diagnosis of cutaneous vascular occlusion syndromes. Adv Dermatol 1999;15(6):153–82.
[19] Asherson RA, Frances C, Iaccarino L, et al. The antiphospholipid antibody syndrome: diagnosis, skin manifestations, and current therapy. Clin Exp Rheumatol 2006;24(Suppl 40): S46–51.
[20] Piette W. Purpura and coagulation. In: Bolognia J, Jorrizo J, Rapini R, editors. Dermatology. 1st edition. London: Mosby; 2003. p. 355–63.
[21] Asherson R. Multiorgan failure and antiphospholipid antibodies: the catastrophic antiphospholipid (Asherson's) syndrome. Immunobiology 2005;210(10):727–33.
[22] Cervera R, Piette JC, Font J, et al. Antiphospholipid syndrome: clinical and immunologic manifestations and patterns of disease expression in a cohort of 1,000 patients. Arthritis Rheum 2002;46(4):1019–27.
[23] Rossini J, Roverano S, Graf C, et al. Widespread cutaneous necrosis associated with antiphospholipid antibodies: report of four cases. J Clin Rheumatol 2002;8(6):326–31.
[24] Pascual J, Gimenez E, Sivera F, et al. Atrophic macules and papules in a 24-year-old woman. Arch Dermatol 2007;143:109–14.
[25] Sparsa A, Piette JC, Weschsler B, et al. Anetoderma and its prothrombotic abnormalities. J Am Acad Dermatol 2003;49(6):1008–12.
[26] Hodak E, Shamai-Lubovitz O, David M, et al. Immunologic abnormalities associated with primary anetoderma. Arch Dermatol 1992;128(6):799–803.
[27] Disdier P, Harle J, Andrac L, et al. Primary anetoderma associated with the antiphospholipid syndrome. J Am Acad Dermatol 1994;30:133–4.

[28] de Souza E, Christofoletti P, Cintra M. Anetoderma associated with primary antiphospholipid syndrome. J Am Acad Dermatol 2007;56(5):881–2.
[29] Venhoff N, Miehle N, Juttner E, et al. Clinical images: anetoderma in systemic lupus erythematosus with antiphospholipid antibodies. Arthritis Rheum 2005;52(7):365–80.
[30] Bilen N, Bayramgurler D, Sikar A, et al. Anetoderma associated with antiphospholipid syndrome and systemic lupus erythematosus. Lupus 2003;12(9):714–6.
[31] Romani J, Perez F, Llobet M, et al. Anetoderma associated with the antiphospholipid antibodies: case report and review of the literature. J Eur Acad Dermatol Venereol 2001;15(2):175–8.

The Role of Antiphospholipid Syndrome in Cardiovascular Disease

Brian R. Long, MD[a],*, Ferdinand Leya, MD[b]

[a]Tennessee Heart & Vascular Institute, P.C., Skyline Medical Center, 3443 Dickerson Pike, Nashville, TN 37207, USA
[b]Cardiac Catheterization Laboratory, Loyola University Medical Center, 2160 South 1st Avenue, Building 107, Room 1858, Maywood, IL 60153, USA

Antiphospholipid antibodies (aPL) are a family of autoantibodies that recognize various phospholipids or phospholipid binding proteins [1]. Lupus anticoagulant antibodies, anticardiolipin antibodies (aCL), and anti-β_2-glycoprotein I (β_2GPI) antibodies are the most commonly detected subgroups of aPL. Patients who have aPL are at risk of developing thrombocytopenia, venous and arterial thrombosis, and recurrent fetal loss [2]. Antiphospholipid syndrome (APS) is defined as the occurrence of these clinical events in association with aPL [3]. Although many cases of APS occur in patients who have systemic lupus erytematosus (SLE), up to 50% of APS patients have primary APS with no underlying systemic disease [4]. It is recognized that aPLs are associated with a spectrum of cardiovascular manifestations including accelerated atherosclerosis, valvular heart disease, intracardiac thrombi, myocardial and pericardial involvement, premature vein graft restenosis, and peripheral vascular disease (Box 1) [5–7]. Furthermore, some studies have demonstrated an association between APS and an increased incidence of myocardial infarction (MI), but this remains controversial. The cardiovascular manifestations of APS will be covered in this article, including recommendations for treatment based on the expert consensus report published in 2003 [8].

CORONARY ARTERY DISEASE IN ANTIPHOSPHOLIPID SYNDROME
Association of Antiphospholipid Antibodies and Atherosclerosis
The prothrombotic state of APS has been implicated in the pathogenesis of premature atherosclerosis in afflicted patients. Although patients who have APS are at higher risk for atherosclerotic cardiovascular events, traditional Framingham risk factors have been shown to be similar between APS patients and the general population [9]. This suggests a direct link between APS and

*Corresponding author. E-mail address: brlong25@hotmail.com (B.R. Long).

> **Box 1: Cardiovascular manifestations of the antiphospholipid syndrome**
>
> *Coronary artery disease*
> Accelerated atherosclerosis
> MI
> Bypass graft failure
> Stent thrombosis
>
> *Valvular disease*
> Nonbacterial vegetations
> Valvular fibrosis and thickening
> Valvular regurgitation
>
> *Cerebral and peripheral arterial occlusion*
> Cardiogenic embolism
> Atherothrombosis in situ
> Paradoxical embolism
>
> *Myocardial dysfunction*
> Diffuse cardiomyopathy
> Diastolic dysfunction
>
> *Intracardiac thrombosis*
> *Pulmonary hypertension*

atherosclerosis. Studies of arterial intima–media thickness (IMT) using B-mode ultrasound in patients with APS have provided evidence for the atherogenic role of these antibodies. Medina and colleagues [10] demonstrated a significant increase in carotid artery IMT with luminal loss among 28 patients with primary APS compared with age- and sex-matched controls. A study by Ames and colleagues [11] examined 42 patients who had aPL, including 29 who had primary APS, and found that IgG aCL titer independently predicted the extent of IMT in all carotid segments examined. Contrary to these results, Vlachoyiannopoulos and colleagues [12] failed to demonstrate an association between aCL or anti-β_2GPI antibodies and atherosclerosis among premenopausal women who had APS and SLE. They did show an increased prevalence of carotid and femoral plaque that was unaccounted for by other traditional risk factors, however.

There is some evidence that all types of aPL are not equal in regards to their potential contribution to thrombosis and atherogenesis. In a retrospective analysis of 637 patients who had APS, Soltesz and colleagues [13] identified differences in the clinical events associated with various types of aPL. Specifically, venous thrombosis occurred more frequently in patients who had lupus anticoagulant, while coronary, carotid, and peripheral artery thrombosis occurred more frequently in subjects who had IgG or IgM aCL. These findings support the association of aPL, specifically antibodies to cardiolipin and its cofactor, β_2-glycoprotein I, with the initiation of atherosclerosis.

Role of Antiphospholipid Antibodies in Atherogenesis

aPLs exert proinflammatory and procoagulant effects directly on endothelial cells, and the inflammatory and immune components of autoantibody-mediated thrombosis may play an indirect role in atherogenesis [9,14]. Antibodies against cardiolipin and endothelial cells have been found among patients with premature atherosclerotic peripheral vascular disease [15]. Vaarala and colleagues [16] first suggested in 1993 that aPL might be involved in atherosclerosis by means of interaction with serum lipoproteins. They found raised concentrations of IgG antibodies to oxidized low-density lipoprotein (LDL) in 80% of patients with SLE, 46% of whom also had elevated levels of IgG aCL antibodies. Furthermore, they reported a cross-reactivity between aCL and antibodies to oxidized LDL, suggesting a potential mechanism for aPL interaction with serum lipoproteins. The presence of autoantibodies directed against serum lipoproteins also was demonstrated in a study by Alves and colleagues [17]. They discovered antibodies directed against high-density lipoprotein (HDL) and Apo A-1 in patients who had SLE and APS, and a high percentage of these antibodies also cross-reacted with aCL.

Antibodies to β_2GPI also have been implicated in atherogenesis. Oxidized LDL forms nondissociable complexes with β_2GPI, and the cross-reaction of autoantibodies against these complexes increases LDL uptake by macrophages, leading to foam cell formation [18,19]. In addition, these autoantibodies can bind β_2GPI on endothelial cells, inducing adhesion molecule expression and thereby contributing to monocyte adherence to the endothelium [20].

Myocardial Infarction and Antiphospholipid Antibodies

Whether there is an association between APS and an increased incidence of MI remains controversial. Elevated levels of aPL first were reported in patients with MI in the 1980s, although it was felt that the rise in antibody titers was a consequence of the acute injury and not indicative of a pathogenic mechanism. Hamsten and colleagues [21] measured aCL levels in 62 patients under age 45 who had survived acute MI. Twenty-one percent of patients had elevated aCL levels, and a higher rate of subsequent cardiovascular events occurred in these patients. A study by Mattila and colleagues [22] showed elevated aCL levels in 15 of 40 acute MI patients compared with one of 41 control patients who had chronic stable coronary artery disease. Zuckerman and colleagues evaluated 124 survivors of acute MI, and found a high prevalence (14%) of positive aCL titers compared with 3% among controls matched for age and coronary risk factors [23]. During the 3-month follow-up period, the rates of thromboembolic events and myocardial reinfarction were significantly higher in the aPL-positive group compared with the aPL-negative group. Conversely, in a cohort of 111 survivors of MI, Raghavan and colleagues [24] found no evidence that patients who had acute or previous MI had higher aPL titers than those found in patients with chronic coronary disease. They also found no correlation of raised aPL titers and post-MI complications.

Bypass Graft Failure and Stent Thrombosis in Antiphospholipid Syndrome

In addition to their association with native coronary artery atherosclerosis and thrombosis, aPLs have been implicated in premature restenosis of vein grafts used in coronary artery bypass surgery (CABG). Morton and colleagues [25] measured aCL titers in 83 patients undergoing CABG, and correlated the results with the incidence of early (1 to 2 weeks) and late (12 months) graft occlusion as determined by angiography. They found a direct correlation between the preoperative antibody level and the incidence of late graft occlusion both in terms of the number of patients with an occlusion and the number of distal anastomotic occlusions. Of the 15 patients who had aCL titers four standard deviations (SD) above mean for controls, eight (53.3 percent) had at least one late graft occlusion. Interestingly, maximum titers that were 2 to 4, 0 to 2, or less than 0 SD above the mean led to late occlusion rates of 23.1%, 9.1%, and 6.7%, respectively. In another study, Bick and colleagues [26] reviewed the cases of 40 patients who had early failure of CABG (15 patients), percutaneous transluminal coronary angioplasty (PTCA) (19 patients), or both (six patients). Of these 40 patients, 12 (30%) were positive for either lupus anticoagulant or aCL.

Stent thrombosis is a rare but serious complication of coronary stenting. When it occurs, cardiologists must evaluate the clinical and technical aspects of the case carefully to better understand the possible causes of stent thrombosis. In some cases, a mechanical problem with stent deployment is at fault, while in others, a previously unrecognized prothrombotic condition is discovered in the patient. Two cases of acute stent thrombosis have been reported in patients with APS. Muir and colleagues [27] described a case of recurrent stent thrombosis that was unexplained by the angiographic appearance of the vessel. The patient later was diagnosed with APS associated with renal cell carcinoma. The second case, reported by Weissman and Coplan [28], was of a 46-year-old woman who had subacute stent thrombosis in three coronary arteries two days after multivessel stenting despite 100% compliance with antiplatelet medications. After repeat PTCA and stenting, the patient developed recurrent ischemia and ultimately required CABG. A thorough evaluation for a hypercoagulable disorder revealed normal levels of proteins C and S, antithrombin III, and homocysteine. Tests for factor V Leiden and prothrombin gene mutations were negative, as were tests for aspirin resistance and clopidogrel resistance. The patient was found to have positive lupus anticoagulant titers, and following CABG, she was discharged on therapeutic warfarin. These cases support the routine screening for aPL in addition to other prothrombotic conditions in patients who experience stent thrombosis. Furthermore, CABG and coronary stenting should be performed with extreme caution in patients who have known APS, and a tailored antiplatelet and anticoagulation regimen is necessary in APS patients requiring these procedures.

VALVE ABNORMALITIES AND PERIPHERAL EMBOLIZATION
Association of Antiphospholipid Syndrome and Valve Disease

Valvular disease was the earliest reported cardiac manifestation of APS [5]. The valvular lesions found in APS are essentially the same entity as SLE-associated Libman-Sacks endocarditis, which classically has been described as verrucous endocarditis of valve leaflets, papillary muscles, and the myocardium (Fig. 1) [29]. The association of aPL with valvular lesions first was recognized in case reports describing nonbacterial vegetations involving the mitral valve in association with cerebral ischemic events in patients who had lupus anticoagulants [30–32]. It now is known that a third to half of patients with primary APS have valve disease, and although it is usually asymptomatic, it can lead to significant mitral and/or aortic regurgitation [33–35]. In addition to valvular thickening and nonbacterial vegetations, actual thrombus formation has been reported on both native and prosthetic heart valves in patients who have APS [36].

The prevalence of aPL in patients who have SLE and heart valve disease has been studied extensively. Leung and colleagues [37] studied 75 patients who had SLE and found that aCL was positive in 23 patients, 16 of whom had echocardiographic abnormalities including verrucous valvular thickening and dysfunction. These abnormalities were statistically more common in aPL-positive patients than in patients without the antibodies. A European multicenter case-controlled study including 132 patients who had SLE found the prevalence of valvular lesions in SLE was 22.7% compared with 2.9% in a group of healthy controls. Fifty of the SLE patients were aPL-positive, and the prevalence of valve vegetations was significantly higher than in aPL-negative SLE

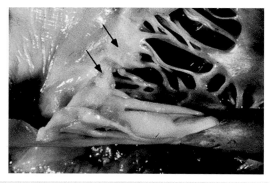

Fig. 1. Libman-Sacks verrucous endocarditis verrucous endocarditis with valvular vegetations (*arrows*) in a 52-year-old woman with systemic lupus erythematosus who died of pneumonia and chronic interstitial pneumonitis. (*Reproduced with permission from* Bermas BL, Erkan D, Schur PH. Clinical manifestations of the antiphospholipid syndrome. In: Rose BD, editor. Waltham (MA): UpToDate;2006. Copyright ©2006 UpToDate Inc. For more information, visit www.uptodate.com.)

patients (16% versus 1.2%, respectively). Mitral regurgitation was present in 38% of aPL-positive patients compared with 12% of patients without aPL, also a statistically significant difference [38].

Primary APS also has been implicated in the development of heart valve disease. Brenner and colleagues [39] performed echocardiograms on 34 patients who had increased levels of serum aCL antibodies with no evidence of malignancy or SLE. They found valvular lesions in 11 of 34 patients (32%), and the lesions were similar to those observed in SLE patients. In a similar study of 28 primary APS patients, Galve and colleagues [40] found valve abnormalities in 10 subjects, all with left-sided valvular regurgitation that was moderate or severe in five cases. Again, valve lesions had the appearance of SLE-associated cardiac disease.

Pathogenesis of Valve Disease in Antiphospholipid Syndrome

The histopathology of aPL-associated valve lesions can show fibrosis, calcification, verrucous superficial thrombosis, intravalvular capillary thrombosis, and vascular proliferation [33,34]. Complement components and immunoglobin deposits including anticardiolipin are common in the diseased valves of patients with both primary and secondary APS [41]. It has been suggested that aPLs interact with antigens on valve surfaces, leading to superficial thrombosis and subendocardial inflammation. These thrombotic and inflammatory changes can lead to the fibrosis and calcification seen in valvulitis [34].

There are several common characteristics linking the heart lesions of rheumatic fever (RF) and the cardiac involvement seen in APS, as summarized by Blank and colleagues [42]. Both diseases can affect the heart and central nervous system. Molecular mimicry between pathogens and autoantigens may occur, with cross-reacting antibodies between the pathogen and self-molecules. In addition, circulating aPLs are found in some patients who have RF, while APS may be associated with streptococcal infection. Recently, a cross-reactivity of antibodies to streptococcal M-protein and antibodies from APS patients targeting β_2GPI was identified. Whether the similarities between RF and APS represent an unlikely coincidence or a true pathogenetic link is a question that requires further investigation.

Thromboembolic Events in Antiphospholipid Antibody-Associated Valve Disease

It is known that aPLs are associated with cerebrovascular occlusions in patients who have SLE and in those who have primary APS. Patients who have SLE or clinical features concerning for APS who present with cerebrovascular events should be screened for these antibodies, as their occurrence may have a bearing on future therapy [43]. APS theoretically can cause cerebral infarction by several mechanisms. These include cardiogenic embolism from nonbacterial vegetations, in situ atherothrombosis by means of endothelial injury of cerebral arteries, and paradoxical embolism of thrombus across the interatrial septum [44]. Bulckaen and colleagues [45] investigated the role of aPL in thromboembolic events and mortality in a prospective cohort study of 89 patients who had severe valvular heart disease. Nineteen subjects had increase aPL titers, and of these, seven (37%) had thromboembolic events during the mean follow-up period of 59 months. Among the 70 aPL-negative patients, eight (11%) had events ($P = .01$). These results suggest that in patients who have severe valvular disease, increased aPL titers portend an increased risk of thromboembolic events.

Association of Antiphospholipid Syndrome and Paradoxical Embolization

Patent foramen ovale (PFO) is a form of atrial septal defect that occurs because of incomplete fusion of the septum primum and septum secundum during embryologic development of the heart. PFO is a common condition, occurring in up to 25% of healthy individuals [46]. Although many patients who have PFO remain asymptomatic throughout their lifetime, complications including cryptogenic stroke can occur. Percutaneous PFO closure is an effective treatment strategy for secondary prevention of paradoxical thromboembolic events that is being used with increasing frequency.

Little is known about the potential interaction between PFO and the various hypercoagulable states associated with cryptogenic stroke [47]. Dodge and colleagues screened 34 consecutive patients undergoing percutaneous PFO closure for several hypercoagulable conditions [47]. In all, 16 patients (47%) had laboratory evidence of arterial hypercoagulability, 13 of whom were aPL-positive (38%). Ago and colleagues [44] described a case of bilateral lower extremity pain and sudden-onset hemianopsia in a 42-year-old woman previously diagnosed with primary APS. She was found to have bilateral femoral vein thrombosis and a right occipital lobe cerebral infarction. Transesophageal echocardiography revealed the presence of PFO with a small right-to-left shunt. The authors concluded that paradoxical embolism through the PFO caused this patient's cerebrovascular accident, and that APS patients should be screened routinely for PFO. This recommendation is supported by the high prevalence of aPL among patients requiring PFO closure for secondary prevention of cerebrovascular events.

MYOCARDIAL INVOLVEMENT IN ANTIPHOSPHOLIPID SYNDROME

Diffuse Cardiomyopathy

There are many common conditions that can affect myocardial function adversely, such as hypertension, valve disease, diabetes mellitus, renal failure, and ischemic heart disease. The presence of these conditions makes the diagnosis of primary myocardial disease a challenge [2]. Among patients who have SLE, there is some evidence that primary myocardial failure may be caused by myocarditis associated with antibodies to ribonucleoproteins and skeletal muscle myositis [48]. There is also evidence suggesting that aPL may play a role in the development of cardiomyopathy in patients who have no other obvious cause such as coronary or valvular disease. In their aforementioned cohort study of 75 SLE patients, Leung and colleagues [37] found elevated aPL levels in four out of the five patients who had isolated left ventricular systolic dysfunction.

Several case reports have demonstrated a possible histopathological explanation for diffuse cardiomyopathy in patients who have aPL. Murphy and Leach [49] described a 33-year-old man with primary APS who died of heart failure. At autopsy, his heart showed widespread thrombosis within the small intramyocardial arterioles, without evidence of vasculitis. In a similar case, Brown and colleagues [50] reported the autopsy findings of a 22-year-old woman with SLE who died of heart failure. Again, there was occlusive microthrombosis of the small arterioles of the heart and other organs. Finally, Kaplan and colleagues [5] reported a young SLE patient who died suddenly from cardiac arrest. The patient had elevated lupus anticoagulant and aCL antibodies, and autopsy revealed a diffuse cardiomyopathy and intramyocardial arteriolar thrombosis without vasculitis. The authors concluded that these findings broaden the spectrum of aPL-associated thrombosis to include small arterioles within the heart. In all three of these cases, there were areas of microinfarction surrounding the affected arterioles, leading to extensive myocardial necrosis. The lack of vasculitic changes on histopathological examination supports the notion of a direct thrombotic effect of aPL rather than a defect in the vessel wall itself.

Diastolic Dysfunction

In addition to diffuse cardiomyopathy causing systolic dysfunction, aPLs have been implicated in primary diastolic dysfunction. Diastolic heart failure is seen commonly in patients who have hypertension, coronary artery disease, and cardiomyopathy. Doppler echocardiography is the diagnostic tool of choice for diastolic dysfunction, and several Doppler parameters are used to evaluate the left ventricular filling pattern for signs of impaired ventricular relaxation. Hasnie and colleagues [51] performed Doppler echocardiography on 10 patients (age range of 20 to 46 years) who had primary APS and 10 healthy controls matched for age, sex, height, and weight. All subjects were free of coronary disease, hypertension, left ventricular hypertrophy, and valvular or pericardial disease that could lead to diastolic heart failure. All four measured parameters of diastolic filling showed a significant association between APS and diastolic dysfunction as compared with the controls. Left ventricular systolic function was normal in all patients, and there was no difference between the groups in regards to left ventricular mass, filling time, or heart rate. It is unclear how aPL might cause impaired diastolic function directly, but diastolic dysfunction frequently precedes systolic failure in other disease states. One therefore could conclude that the abnormal left ventricular filling pattern seen in patients who have APS may be an early manifestation of myocardial involvement.

INTRACARDIAC THROMBOSIS

Thrombus formation on the endocardial surface is a rare but important cardiac manifestation of aPL. Reports of primary intracardiac mural thrombi occurring in all four heart chambers have been published [5,52–54]. Leventhal and colleagues [53] reported a right atrial thrombus in a young male with recurrent deep venous thrombosis and thrombocytopenia. This patient had positive lupus anticoagulant and aCL IgG antibodies. The location and echocardiographic appearance of this mass mimicked a typical right atrial myxoma. The surgical findings, however, were of a thrombus attached to the atrial wall with no underlying cardiac abnormality. Kaplan and colleagues [5] were the first to report a left ventricular thrombus in a patient with aPL. They described a 38-year-old female with SLE who presented with fever and confusion. Echocardiography revealed a large mobile apical thrombus, normal valves, and decreased left ventricular systolic function. The patient subsequently suffered a massive stroke despite anticoagulation with heparin, and on repeat echocardiography, the thrombus was no longer present. This patient had elevated levels of aCL IgG and IgM antibodies. Although severe ventricular dysfunction itself can be associated with left ventricular thrombus, the reports of primary intracardiac thrombosis in other cardiac chambers suggest a possible contribution of aPL in this case. Regardless of their etiology, all cases of intracardiac thrombosis require intensive systemic anticoagulation, as discussed later in this article.

PULMONARY HYPERTENSION

The development of pulmonary hypertension (PHT) is a relatively common and sometimes devastating complication of connective tissue diseases such as progressive systemic sclerosis (CREST syndrome) and SLE. Among patients who have SLE, the prevalence of clinically evident PHT is 1% to 14% [55]. In lupus patients, PHT often occurs in the setting of pulmonary vasculitis and/or interstitial lung disease that may lead to elevated pulmonary vascular resistance [8]. Alternatively, SLE-associated aPL may play a role in the development of PHT. Petri and colleagues [56] studied 60 consecutive SLE patients and found an association between positive lupus anticoagulant titers and an increased frequency of PHT. The mechanism by which circulating aPL may lead to PHT is assumed to be recurrent pulmonary embolism, or chronic thromboembolic PHT [8]. This is an infrequent cause of PHT, occurring in 0.1% to 0.2% of patients who survive an acute venous thromboembolic event [57].

Patients who have primary APS also can develop a broad spectrum of pulmonary complications, the most common of which are pulmonary thromboembolism and PHT. Microvascular pulmonary thrombosis, pulmonary capillaritis, and alveolar hemorrhage also have been reported in patients who have APS. Among medical patients with chronic thromboembolic PHT, the prevalence of aPL varies between 10% and 50% [58]. To determine the prevalence of hypercoagulable states among patients with chronic thromboembolic PHT, Colorio and colleagues [57] retrospectively analyzed 24 patients with the condition and determined the frequency of various thrombophilic risk factors that had been measured in some or all patients. A positive aPL titer was the most common abnormality found, occurring in 12 of 24 patients. Among patients checked for other hypercoagulable states, 7 of 14 had hyperhomocysteinemia. One of 10 had protein S deficiency; 1 of 13 had protein C deficiency, and activated protein C resistance was found in 1 of 22 patients. Additionally, antithrombin III deficiency was found in 1 of 24 patients, and prothrombin gene mutation was found in 1 of 18 patients studied. Interestingly, factor V Leiden was normal in all 18 patients tested. In total, 75% of patients who had chronic thromboembolic PHT had at least one thrombophilic risk factor, the most common being aPL, which occurred in 50% of cases. These findings support the routine screening for thrombophilic states in patients who have chronic thromboembolic PHT. In addition, clinicians seriously should consider the various types of aPL-associated vascular injury when evaluating APS patients who present with dyspnea, fever, and infiltrates on chest radiography [58].

TREATMENT OF CARDIOVASCULAR DISEASE IN ANTIPHOSPHOLIPID SYNDROME

In 2003, a 10-member expert committee published a consensus report of recommendations for treatment of cardiac disease in APS [8]. This report covered five major cardiovascular sequelae of the disease, as summarized in Table 1. The committee's recommendations and the data supporting their rationale are presented in this section.

Coronary Artery Disease

Patients who have APS should be screened and treated for all traditional coronary artery disease risk factors including hypertension, hypercholesterolemia, smoking, and diabetes. The LDL-lowering drugs known as HMG-CoA inhibitors, or statins, are known to cause a regression of atherosclerotic lesions and a reduction of cardiovascular complications [59,60]. Furthermore, statin drugs have been shown to decrease cardiovascular events regardless of pretreatment cholesterol levels, suggesting a non-LDL effect of the drug class on atherosclerotic disease [61]. One possible mechanism for the antiatherosclerotic effects of statins involves the anti-β_2GPI-induced proadhesive and proinflammatory endothelial phenotype. Meroni and colleagues [62] demonstrated that endothelial activation mediated by anti-β_2GPI antibodies can be inhibited by statins. Given the suggested role of endothelial activation in aPL-related atherogenesis, statins may be especially useful for preventing atherosclerotic disease in patients who have APS.

In addition to statins, hydroxychloroquine was shown to provide protective cardiovascular effects in the Hopkins Lupus Cohort [63]. The positive effects of hydroxychloroquine are probably multifactorial, including suppression of active SLE, a reduction in aPL, antiplatelet effects, and lipid-lowering effects [8]. Finally, elevated plasma homocysteine may be implicated in APS-related arterial thrombosis [8], suggesting a possible role for folic acid supplementation in patients who have APS. Based on these findings, the committee recommended liberal use of statins in all patients who have APS, plus consideration of folic acid, B vitamins, and hydroxychloroquine for cardiac protection in

Table 1
Summary of panel findings and recommendations

Abnormality	Prevalence of pAPS	Prevalence of sAPS	Strength of data	Panel treatment consensus
Valve disease	35% to 50%	35% to 50%	Many TTE and TEE studies	Stroke prophylaxis for symptomatic patients (for asymptomatic patients, a survey of experts recommends aspirin); theoretical basis for immunosuppression; distinguish among valvulitis, valve deformity, and vegetation in clinical trials
Coronary occlusion	5%	5.9%	Population studies primarily of patients who have systemic lupus erythematosus (SLE)	Aggressive treatment of atherosclerosis and its risk factors; anticoagulation (warfarin) for documented thrombosis; consider hydroxychloroquine, statins
Ventricular dysfunction	No reliable figures	23% to 32% in SLE; no reliable figures for sAPS	Case series, not segregated by antiphospholipid syndrome status; SLE population studies	No known effective treatment; no recommendations
Intracardiac thrombi	No reliable figures	No reliable figures	Case reports	Anticoagulation with warfarin; possible surgical excision
Pulmonary hypertension	1% to 3%	4% (symptomatic; up to 14% asymptomatic)	Population studies of TTE	Anticoagulation with warfarin; consider bosentan, epoprostenol

Abbreviations: pAPS, primary antiphospholipid syndrome; sAPS, secondary antiphospholipid syndrome; TTE, transthoracic echocardiography; TEE, transesophageal echocardiography.
Adapted from Lockshin M, Tenedios F, Petri M, et al. Cardiac disease in the antiphospholipid syndrome: recommendations for treatment. Committee consensus report. Lupus 2003;12(7):518–23; with permission.

patients at elevated cardiovascular risk. For patients who develop arterial thrombosis in the absence of atherosclerotic disease, prolonged anticoagulation with warfarin is recommended [64].

Treatment of Valve Abnormalities in Antiphospholipid Syndrome

As described in the section on valvular disease, there are several pathological changes that can occur in patients who have APS, including valvulitis with thickening, valve deformity and failure, and vegetation formation. Unfortunately, many of the publications about the prevalence and pathogenesis of valve disease in APS do not clearly delineate between these different entities, making recommendations for treatment somewhat challenging. A study by Espnola-Zavaleta and colleagues [65] provided some insight into the utility of antiplatelet and anticoagulant therapy in APS patients with valvular disease. They performed transesophageal echocardiograms (TEE) on 13 primary APS patients before starting aspirin and/or warfarin therapy, and then repeated the test after 12 months of treatment. They found no modification of valve lesions in six cases (46.2%), with the remaining seven patients (53.8%) developing new lesions. The authors concluded that oral antiplatelet or anticoagulation therapy does not diminish the noninfective valve lesions seen in primary APS. There is also controversy over the use of corticosteroids or other anti-inflammatory drugs to treat valvular disease in primary or secondary APS. To date, there are no published systematic studies on anti-inflammatory or immunosuppressive treatment for this condition [8].

Because of the increased risk of systemic embolization from vegetations and valve thickening, the committee recommends anticoagulation with warfarin or heparin for APS patients with documented valvulopathy and any evidence of thromboembolic disease. They also support the prophylactic use of antiplatelet therapy for asymptomatic patients. No agreement, however, was reached regarding corticosteroid treatment for acute valve inflammation.

Myocardial Involvement in Antiphospholipid Syndrome

Because of the lack of published studies addressing treatment of this manifestation of APS, it is unknown whether antiplatelet, anticoagulant, or other treatment may be useful in preventing the diffuse cardiomyopathy or diastolic dysfunction seen in patients who have APS [8]. Therefore, the committee made no recommendations on this condition. Standard medical therapy for systolic or diastolic heart failure should be initiated and optimized according to current treatment guidelines.

Intracardiac Thrombosis

In case reports of intracardiac thrombi in patients who have APS, physicians have described treatment strategies of aggressive anticoagulation and/or surgical incision. There are no published studies comparing medical, surgical, or combined treatment strategies for this complication of APS. The committee's recommendations were to screen patients who have APS for intracardiac thrombosis, initiate intensive warfarin anticoagulation when thrombus is identified, and to consult cardiac surgeons when appropriate.

Pulmonary Hypertension

As described previously, recurrent pulmonary embolism is the presumed cause of PHT in APS. Treatment, therefore, is directed at preventing and treating venous thromboembolic disease. Acute pulmonary embolism requires treatment with heparin followed by warfarin, and long-term warfarin is indicated for prophylactic treatment of recurrent pulmonary embolism with or without APS. The appropriate therapeutic range for the international normalized ratio (INR) remains controversial, but an intensive, closely monitored treatment plan is recommended. Other treatments for PHT, including calcium channel blockers, bosentan, cyclophosphamide, and intravenous prostacyclin or eporostenol infusions, have not been studied specifically in PHT associated with APS.

SUMMARY

APS is associated with various cardiovascular abnormalities. A link between APS and atherosclerosis of peripheral and coronary arteries has been established, and the role of aPL in atherogenesis is becoming clearer as researchers uncover the cellular and molecular mechanisms of the disease. Valvular heart disease was the first reported cardiac manifestation of APS, with pathological findings ranging from verrucous endocarditis with nonbacterial vegetations to valvular thickening and insufficiency. Less frequently, APS has been associated with myocardial dysfunction in the form of diffuse primary cardiomyopathy or impaired relaxation causing diastolic heart failure. Intracardiac thrombosis and pulmonary hypertension also have been associated with APS, and they always should be considered in APS patients presenting with the appropriate clinical signs and symptoms. This article reviewed the prevalence and proposed mechanisms of these various cardiovascular diseases associated with APS, and concluded with a discussion of current recommendations for treatment.

References

[1] Levine JS, Branch DW, Rauch J. The antiphospholipid syndrome [see comment]. N Engl J Med 2002;346(10):752–63.

[2] Asherson RA, Cervera R. Antiphospholipid antibodies and the heart. Lessons and pitfalls for the cardiologist [see comment]. Circulation 1991;84(2):920–3.

[3] Sammaritano LR, Gharavi AE, Lockshin MD. Antiphospholipid antibody syndrome: immunologic and clinical aspects. Semin Arthritis Rheum 1990;20(2):81–96.

[4] Godfrey T, D'cruz D. Antiphospholipid syndrome: general features. In: Khamashta M, editor. Hughes syndrome. Antiphospholipid syndrome. London: Springer; 2000. p. 8–19.

[5] Kaplan SD, Chartash EK, Pizzarello RA, et al. Cardiac manifestations of the antiphospholipid syndrome. Am Heart J 1992;124(5):1331–8.

[6] Puisieux F, de Groote P, Masy E, et al. Association between anticardiolipin antibodies and mortality in patients with peripheral arterial disease. Am J Med 2000;109(8):635–41.

[7] Shoenfeld Y, Gerli R, Doria A, et al. Accelerated atherosclerosis in autoimmune rheumatic diseases. Circulation 2005;112(21):3337–47.

[8] Lockshin M, Tenedios F, Petri M, et al. Cardiac disease in the antiphospholipid syndrome: recommendations for treatment. Committee consensus report. Lupus 2003;12(7):518–23.
[9] Jara LJ, Medina G, Vera-Lastra O, et al. Atherosclerosis and antiphospholipid syndrome. Clin Rev Allergy Immunol 2003;25(1):79–88.
[10] Medina G, Casaos D, Jara LJ, et al. Increased carotid artery intima–media thickness may be associated with stroke in primary antiphospholipid syndrome [see comment]. Ann Rheum Dis 2003;62(7):607–10.
[11] Ames PR, Margarita A, Delgado Alves J, et al. Anticardiolipin antibody titre and plasma homocysteine level independently predict intima media thickness of carotid arteries in subjects with idiopathic antiphospholipid antibodies. Lupus 2002;11(4):208–14.
[12] Vlachoyiannopoulos PG, Kanellopoulos PG, Ioannidis JP, et al. Atherosclerosis in premenopausal women with antiphospholipid syndrome and systemic lupus erythematosus: a controlled study. Rheumatology (Oxford) 2003;42(5):645–51.
[13] Soltesz P, Veres K, Lakos G, et al. Evaluation of clinical and laboratory features of antiphospholipid syndrome: a retrospective study of 637 patients. Lupus 2003;12(4):302–7.
[14] Shoenfeld Y, Harats D, George J. Atherosclerosis and the antiphospholipid syndrome: a link unravelled? Lupus 1998;7(Suppl 2):S140–3.
[15] Nityanand S, Bergmark C, de Faire U, et al. Antibodies against endothelial cells and cardiolipin in young patients with peripheral atherosclerotic disease [see comment]. J Intern Med 1995;238(5):437–43.
[16] Vaarala O, Alfthan G, Jauhiainen M, et al. Cross-reaction between antibodies to oxidised low-density lipoprotein and to cardiolipin in systemic lupus erythematosus. Lancet 1993;341(8850):923–5.
[17] Delgado Alves J, Kumar S, Isenberg DA. Cross-reactivity between anti-cardiolipin, anti-high-density lipoprotein and antiapolipoprotein A-I IgG antibodies in patients with systemic lupus erythematosus and primary antiphospholipid syndrome. Rheumatology (Oxford) 2003;42(7):893–9.
[18] Kobayashi K, Kishi M, Atsumi T, et al. Circulating oxidized LDL forms complexes with beta2-glycoprotein I: implication as an atherogenic autoantigen. J Lipid Res 2003;44(4):716–26.
[19] van Leuven SI, Kastelein JJ, D'Cruz DP, et al. Atherogenesis in rheumatology. Lupus 2006;15(3):117–21.
[20] Matsuura E, Koike T. Accelerated atheroma and anti-beta2-glycoprotein I antibodies. Lupus 2000;9(3):210–6.
[21] Hamsten A, Norberg R, Bjorkholm M, et al. Antibodies to cardiolipin in young survivors of myocardial infarction: an association with recurrent cardiovascular events. Lancet 1986;1(8473):113–6.
[22] Mattila K, Vaarala O, Palosuo T, et al. Serologic response against cardiolipin and enterobacterial common antigen in young patients with acute myocardial infarction. Clin Immunol Immunopathol 1989;51(3):414–8.
[23] Zuckerman E, Toubi E, Shiran A, et al. Anticardiolipin antibodies and acute myocardial infarction in nonsystemic lupus erythmatosus patients: a controlled prospective study [see comment]. Am J Med 1996;101(4):381–6.
[24] Raghavan C, Ditchfield J, Taylor RJ, et al. Influence of anticardiolipin antibodies on immediate patient outcome after myocardial infarction. J Clin Pathol 1993;46(12):1113–5.
[25] Morton KE, Gavaghan TP, Krilis SA, et al. Coronary artery bypass graft failure—an autoimmune phenomenon? [erratum appears in Lancet 1987 Oct 24;2(8565):977–8]. Lancet 1986;2(8520):1353–7.
[26] Bick RL, Ismail Y, Baker WF Jr. Coagulation abnormalities in patients with precocious coronary artery thrombosis and patients failing coronary artery bypass grafting and percutaneous transcoronary angioplasty. Semin Thromb Hemost 1993;19(4):412–7.
[27] Muir DF, Stevens A, Napier-Hemy RO, et al. Recurrent stent thrombosis associated with lupus anticoagulant due to renal cell carcinoma. Int J Cardiovasc Intervent 2003;5(1):44–6.

[28] Weissman A, Coplan N. Antiphospholipid antibody syndrome and acute stent thrombosis. Rev Cardiovasc Med 2006;7(4):244–6.
[29] Libman E, Sacks B. A hitherto undescribed form of valvular and mural endocarditis. Arch Intern Med 1924;33:701–37.
[30] Anderson D, Bell D, Lodge R, et al. Recurrent cerebral ischemia and mitral valve vegetation in a patient with antiphospholipid antibodies. J Rheumatol 1987;14(4):839–41.
[31] D'Alton JG, Preston DN, Bormanis J, et al. Multiple transient ischemic attacks, lupus anticoagulant, and verrucous endocarditis. Stroke 1985;16(3):512–4.
[32] Ford SE, Lillicrap D, Brunet D, et al. Thrombotic endocarditis and lupus anticoagulant. A pathogenetic possibility for idiopathic rheumatic type valvular heart disease. Arch Pathol Lab Med 1989;113(4):350–3.
[33] Cervera R. Recent advances in antiphospholipid antibody-related valvulopathies. J Autoimmun 2000;15(2):123–5.
[34] Nesher G, Ilany J, Rosenmann D, et al. Valvular dysfunction in antiphospholipid syndrome: prevalence, clinical features, and treatment. Semin Arthritis Rheum 1997;27(1):27–35.
[35] Chartash EK, Lans DM, Paget SA, et al. Aortic insufficiency and mitral regurgitation in patients with systemic lupus erythematosus and the antiphospholipid syndrome. Am J Med 1989;86(4):407–12.
[36] Ford PM, Ford SE, Lillicrap DP. Association of lupus anticoagulant with severe valvular heart disease in systemic lupus erythematosus. J Rheumatol 1988;15(4):597–600.
[37] Leung WH, Wong KL, Lau CP, et al. Association between antiphospholipid antibodies and cardiac abnormalities in patients with systemic lupus erythematosus. Am J Med 1990;89(4):411–9.
[38] Khamashta MA, Cervera R, Asherson RA, et al. Association of antibodies against phospholipids with heart valve disease in systemic lupus erythematosus [see comment]. Lancet 1990;335(8705):1541–4.
[39] Brenner B, Blumenfeld Z, Markiewicz W, et al. Cardiac involvement in patients with primary antiphospholipid syndrome. J Am Coll Cardiol 1991;18(4):931–6.
[40] Galve E, Ordi J, Barquinero J, et al. Valvular heart disease in the primary antiphospholipid syndrome. Ann Intern Med 1992;116(4):293–8.
[41] Ziporen L, Goldberg I, Arad M, et al. Libman-Sacks endocarditis in the antiphospholipid syndrome: immunopathologic findings in deformed heart valves. Lupus 1996;5(3):196–205.
[42] Blank M, Aron-Maor A, Shoenfeld Y. From rheumatic fever to Libman-Sacks endocarditis: is there any possible pathogenetic link? Lupus 2005;14(9):697–701.
[43] Asherson RA, Khamashta MA, Gil A, et al. Cerebrovascular disease and antiphospholipid antibodies in systemic lupus erythematosus, lupus-like disease, and the primary antiphospholipid syndrome [see comment]. Am J Med 1989;86(4):391–9.
[44] Ago T, Ooboshi H, Kitazono T, et al. Brain infarction associated with antiphospholipid antibody syndrome caused by paradoxical embolism through patent foramen ovale [see comment]. J Neurol 2004;251(6):757–9.
[45] Bulckaen HG, Puisieux FL, Bulckaen ED, et al. Antiphospholipid antibodies and the risk of thromboembolic events in valvular heart disease. Mayo Clin Proc 2003;78(3):294–8.
[46] Meissner I, Whisnant JP, Khandheria BK, et al. Prevalence of potential risk factors for stroke assessed by transesophageal echocardiography and carotid ultrasonography: the SPARC study. Stroke prevention: assessment of risk in a community [see comment]. Mayo Clin Proc 1999;74(9):862–9.
[47] Dodge SM, Hassell K, Anderson CA, et al. Antiphospholipid antibodies are common in patients referred for percutaneous patent foramen ovale closure. Catheter Cardiovasc Interv 2004;61(1):123–7.
[48] Borenstein DG, Fye WB, Arnett FC, et al. The myocarditis of systemic lupus erythematosus: association with myositis. Ann Intern Med 1978;89(5 Pt 1):619–24.
[49] Murphy JJ, Leach IH. Findings at necropsy in the heart of a patient with anticardiolipin syndrome. Br Heart J 1989;62(1):61–4.

[50] Brown JH, Doherty CC, Allen DC, et al. Fatal cardiac failure due to myocardial microthrombi in systemic lupus erythematosus. Br Med J (Clin Res Ed) 1988;296(6635):1505.
[51] Hasnie AM, Stoddard MF, Gleason CB, et al. Diastolic dysfunction is a feature of the antiphospholipid syndrome. Am Heart J 1995;129(5):1009–13.
[52] Coppock MA, Safford RE, Danielson GK. Intracardiac thrombosis, phospholipid antibodies, and two-chambered right ventricle. Br Heart J 1988;60(5):455–8.
[53] Leventhal LJ, Borofsky MA, Bergey PD, et al. Antiphospholipid antibody syndrome with right atrial thrombosis mimicking an atrial myxoma. Am J Med 1989;87(1):111–3.
[54] Lubbe WF, Asherson RA. Intracardiac thrombus in systemic lupus erythematosus associated with lupus anticoagulant. Arthritis Rheum 1988;31(11):1453–4.
[55] Petri M. Systemic lupus erythematosis and the cardiovascular system: the heart. In: Lahita R, editor. Systemic lupus erythematosis. 3rd edition. San Diego: Academic Press; 1999. p. 687–706.
[56] Petri M, Rheinschmidt M, Whiting-O'Keefe Q, et al. The frequency of lupus anticoagulant in systemic lupus erythematosus. A study of sixty consecutive patients by activated partial thromboplastin time, Russell viper venom time, and anticardiolipin antibody level. Ann Intern Med 1987;106(4):524–31.
[57] Colorio CC, Martinuzzo ME, Forastiero RR, et al. Thrombophilic factors in chronic thromboembolic pulmonary hypertension. Blood Coagul Fibrinolysis 2001;12(6):427–32.
[58] Espinosa G, Cervera R, Font J, et al. The lung in the antiphospholipid syndrome. Ann Rheum Dis 2002;61(3):195–8.
[59] Cannon CP, Braunwald E, McCabe CH, et al. Intensive versus moderate lipid lowering with statins after acute coronary syndromes [see comment] [erratum appears in N Engl J Med 2006 Feb 16;354(7):778]. N Engl J Med 2004;350(15):1495–504.
[60] Nissen SE, Tuzcu EM, Schoenhagen P, et al. Effect of intensive compared with moderate lipid-lowering therapy on progression of coronary atherosclerosis: a randomized controlled trial [see comment]. JAMA 2004;291(9):1071–80.
[61] Collins R, Armitage J, Parish S, et al. MRC/BHF Heart protection study of cholesterol lowering with simvastatin in 20,536 high-risk individuals: a randomised placebo-controlled trial. Lancet 2002;360(9326):7–22.
[62] Meroni PL, Raschi E, Testoni C, et al. Statins prevent endothelial cell activation induced by antiphospholipid (anti-beta2-glycoprotein I) antibodies: effect on the proadhesive and proinflammatory phenotype. Arthritis Rheum 2001;44(12):2870–8.
[63] Petri M. Detection of coronary artery disease and the role of traditional risk factors in the Hopkins Lupus Cohort. Lupus 2000;9(3):170–5.
[64] Ruiz-Irastorza G, Khamashta MA, Hunt BJ, et al. Bleeding and recurrent thrombosis in definite antiphospholipid syndrome: analysis of a series of 66 patients treated with oral anticoagulation to a target international normalized ratio of 3.5. Arch Intern Med 2002;162(10):1164–9.
[65] Espinola-Zavaleta N, Vargas-Barron J, Colmenares-Galvis T, et al. Echocardiographic evaluation of patients with primary antiphospholipid syndrome. Am Heart J 1999;137(5):973–8.

Antiphospholipid Syndrome: Role of Antiphospholipid Antibodies in Neurology

Rima M. Dafer, MD, MPH, FAHA*,
José Biller, MD, FACP, FAAN, FAHA

Department of Neurology, Loyola University Chicago,
Stritch School of Medicine, 2160 South First Avenue, 2700 McGuire,
Maywood, IL 60153, USA

Antiphospholipid syndrome (APS), or Hughes syndrome, is an acquired prothrombotic syndrome first described in 1983, characterized by recurrent arterial or venous thromboembolism, unexplained fetal loss usually within the first 10 weeks of gestation, and thrombocytopenia, with the presence of circulating antiphospholipid antibodies.

Primary APS is an immune-mediated coagulopathy associated with cerebral ischemia in young adults, the etiology of which remains unknown. Secondary APS can occur within the context of several diseases, mainly autoimmune or rheumatologic disorders, infections, malignancy, and drugs.

Although only ischemic stroke is reasonably well established and accepted neurological diagnostic criterion for the syndrome, other neurological conditions have been associated with aPLs, most commonly multiple sclerosis, migraine, psychiatric diseases, and various movement disorders.

ANTIPHOSPHOLIPID ANTIBODIES

The antiphospholipid antibodies (aPLs) are antibodies directed against protein antigens that bind to membrane anionic phospholipids, anticardiolipins, or their associated plasma proteins [1]. Several aPLs have been described; the most thoroughly studied subsets include lupus anticoagulant (LA) and anticardiolipin (aCL) IgG, IgA, and IgM isotypes; antiphospahtidylethanolamine (aPE); antiphospatidylserine (aPS); and antiphospathylcholine (aPC). Binding of aCL to cell membrane requires the presence of beta-2 glycoprotein 1 antibody (β2GP1) [2] and prothrombin [3]. LA often is found in patients who have systemic lupus erythematosus (SLE) and in sera from patients who have syphilis binding to cardiolipin extracts of beef hearts. LA is identified by prolonged clotting time on coagulation assays. In contrast, aCLs and

*Corresponding author. E-mail address: rdafer@lumc.edu (R.M. Dafer).

β2GP1 are identified by solid-phase ELISAs that measure immunoreactivity to a phospholipid or phospholipid-binding protein.

EPIDEMIOLOGY

The aPL titers tend to be nonspecific; they are present in 1% to 5% of healthy individuals, and 12% to 50% of elderly patients and patients who have SLE [4–6]. In the Framingham original cohort and offspring combined, the prevalence of aCL positivity was 19.7% in men and 17.6% in women, and was higher in subjects of both genders with first ischemic stroke or transient ischemic attack (TIA) [7]. Familial incidence has been reported in 33% of subjects.

The primary APS affects predominantly younger adults of both genders, with female predominance, although it has been reported in extremes of age. The syndrome is common among all ethnicities, with higher prevalence in African Americans and the Hispanic population. LA appears to be the stronger predictor of thrombotic risk for both venous and arterial thrombosis with an odds ratio of thrombosis five to 16 times higher than control [8,9], followed by anti- β2GP1 antibodies, which correlate mainly with arterial thrombosis. The aCLs are the weakest predictors of thrombosis, correlating mainly with venous rather than arterial thrombosis. The presence of multiple aPLs is thought to carry a higher risk of thrombosis.

PATHOPHYSIOLOGY

The IgG isotypes of aCL and LA are the mostly associated aPLs with risk for first ischemic stroke. The real underlying mechanism of thrombosis remains unclear. Several mechanisms have been postulated, including multifactorial interactions with phospholipids in endothelial cells and platelet membranes, multifactorial interactions with coagulation factors, direct abrogation of endothelial cell prostacyclin production, and down-regulation of interleukins in vascular beds.

CLASSIFICATION CRITERIA FOR ANTIPHOSPHOLIPID SYNDROME

The preliminary Sapporo classification divided the APS criteria into clinical and laboratory, with a definite diagnosis considered when at least one of the clinical and one of the laboratory criteria are present [10]. The criteria were revised at the 11th International Congress on Antiphospholipid Antibodies in Sydney, Australia, in 2004. According to the updated classification, definite diagnosis of APS requires the combination of at least one clinical and one laboratory criterion; the autoantibodies must be detected on at least 2 occasions, 12 weeks apart, to distinguish persistent autoimmune antibody responses from transient responses caused by other conditions such as infection or drug exposures. The diagnosis of APS should be avoided if less than 12 weeks or more than 5 years separate the positive aPL test and the clinical manifestation [11].

The following revised criteria were suggested for the classification of the antiphospholipid syndrome (Box 1).

> **Box 1: Criteria for classifying antiphospholipid syndrome**
>
> *Thrombotic events*
> One or more arterial or venous thrombotic event (VTE) in small vessel in any tissue or organ, in the absence of vasculitis.
>
> *Pregnancy morbidity*
> One or more unexplained fetal loss beyond the 10th week of gestation, or
> At least one premature birth at or before the 34th week of gestation because of eclampsia or pre-eclampsia, or severe placental insufficiency, or
> Three or more unexplained consecutive spontaneous abortions before the 10th week of gestation, with other causes excluded
>
> *Laboratory criteria*
> IgG and/or IgM aCLs in moderately high titers (greater than 40 immunoglobulin G plasma level) in serum or plasma on at least two occasions at least 12 weeks apart by standardized ELISA
> Anti- β2GP1of IgG and/or IgM isotypes in serum or plasma on at least two occasions at least 12 weeks apart measured by a standardized ELISA
> Positive LA in plasma on at least occasions at least 12 weeks apart in the absence of other coagulopathies

Conditions commonly associated with APS not included in the revised criteria include thrombocytopenia, livedo reticularis, heart valve disease, nephropathy, nonischemic neurological manifestations, IgA aCL, IgA anti-β2GP1, aPEs, aPSs, antibodies against prothrombin alone, and antibodies to phospatidylserine–prothrombin complex.

CLINICAL PRESENTATIONS

In addition to cerebral infarctions, arterial or VTEs may involve any tissue or organ in patients who have APS. Coronary artery events are common, accounting for 25% of arterial thrombosis, second only to cerebral infarctions. Retinal thrombosis, adrenal gland infarction or hemorrhage, peripheral venous thrombosis, pulmonary embolism and pulmonary hypertension, myocardial infarction, and skin infarction mainly in patients receiving warfarin therapy, may occur. Other features include recurrent miscarriage, thrombocytopenia, livedo reticularis, renal and celiac artery stenosis, ischemic bone fractures, and avascular necrosis of bone.

Anticardiolipin antibodies increasingly are recognized as important risk factors for cerebral ischemia, especially in young patients [12–16], and are thought to be an independent risk factor for first ischemic stroke [17–21], with one study suggesting a fourfold increased risk of ischemic stroke in patients who have circulating IgG aCL [19]. Other cohort studies have shown that high titers do not correlate with stroke recurrence [13]. A high prevalence of aPLs of 44% was demonstrated in young adult patients under the age of 51 with cerebral ischemia of undetermined causes [22,23]. The prevalence of the disorder, however, is variable because of heterogeneity of aPL, variability and lack of specificity of the assays, and the change in the status of aPL from positive to negative with time. Whether the presence of aPL plays a direct role in stroke or whether it is an epiphenomenon remains unclear, but it is postulated that the presence of circulating aPLs may cause a possible tendency toward accelerated atherosclerosis. Prospective studies have found an association between aPLs and stroke [24], in particular in young adult women [25]. In the antiphospholipid antibodies and stroke study (APASS), the risk of cerebral infarction was reported to be 2.31 times higher in patients who have positive circulating antibodies than in those negative for antibodies [17], but the presence of aPLs (either LA or aCL) among patients who had ischemic stroke did not predict either increased risk of subsequent vascular occlusive events over 2 years or a differential response to antiaggregants [26]. In the Framingham study, elevated serum concentrations of aCLs, independently of other cardiovascular risk factors, significantly predicted the risk of future ischemic stroke and TIA in women but not in men [7]. In the Honolulu study, the risk of stroke and myocardial infarction was 1.5 times higher in men who had positive $\beta 2GP1$-dependent aCL IgG [24].

The most common cerebral ischemia associated with aPLs is arterial infarction, with small vessels and the middle cerebral arteries being the most involved in the arterial circulation. Multiple recurrent cerebral infarctions may occur [27]. Cerebral vein or dural sinus thrombosis are not uncommon.

Although the neurological association of aPLs and APS is diverse, only ischemic stroke is established reasonably well and accepted as a diagnostic criterion for the syndrome. A wide spectrum of neurological disorders, including seizures [28], psychiatric diseases [29], dementia [30], transverse myelitis [31,32], optic neuropathy and multiple sclerosis-like disorders [33–35], migraine [36,37], Guillain-Barré syndrome [38], sensory-neural hearing loss [39–42], and atypical movement disorders, most commonly chorea, hemidystonia, parkinsonism, and hemiballismus, also has been associated with positive aPLs [43] or APS [42].

Dermatological manifestations are encountered in 50% of patients and may be the presenting features in 30.5% of patients. The most frequent dermatological manifestation is livedo reticularis (livedo racemosa), observed in 25.5% of patients. Painful purpura and leg ulcers also may occur. The presence of livedo reticularis is significantly associated with cerebral or ocular ischemic arterial events and Sneddon's syndrome [44].

Cardiac involvement is common in APS, and is related significantly to high IgG aCL titers [45]. Coronary artery disease, mitral valve thickening and other cardiac valvulopathies, and embolic sources frequently are observed. Splinter hemorrhages and cardiac murmur rarely may be seen in patients who have Libman Sacks endocarditis. The use of platelet antiaggregants did not prevented valvular lesion regression in patients who had APS [45]. In patients who have pulmonary embolism, tachypnea and chest pain are common.

Funduscopic examination may show retinal artery occlusion or retinal veins thrombosis. Gangrene of distal extremities and digital ulcers may be present.

CATASTROPHIC ANTIPHOSPHOLIPID SYNDROME
Catastrophic APS or Asherson's syndrome is a life-threatening condition that occurs in less than 1% of patients who have APS. The syndrome is characterized by fulminant thrombotic complications predominantly affecting small vessels, multiple organs involvement, with subsequent multi-organ failure and potentially lethal outcome. An international registry of patients with catastrophic APS, (CAPS Registry), was created in 2000 by the European Forum on Antiphospholipid Antibodies. So far, the registry has included extensive clinical, laboratory, and therapeutic data on approximately 300 patients. Malignancy and/or surgical procedures often were the triggering factors for the disorder [46]. Cerebral manifestations were the most common, predominantly cerebral infarction, followed by encephalopathy [47]. Death occurred in 44% of patients [48]. The leading causes of death in catastrophic patients who had catastrophic APS were from cerebral involvement, mainly cerebral infarctions, followed by cardiac involvement and infections [49]. The presence of SLE was associated with higher mortality rate [50], while higher recovery rate was associated with combined treatment with anticoagulation and corticosteroids plus plasma exchange and/or intravenous immunoglobulins [48]. Unlike patients who had SLE, concomitant treatment with cyclophosphamide did not demonstrate additional benefit in patients who had primary catastrophic APS [50].

CAUSES
The etiology of APS remains unknown. APS is an autoimmune disorder, probably triggered by infections such as syphilis, hepatitis C, HIV, malaria, and septicemia, and by certain drugs including procainamide, propranolol, hydralazine, quinine, phenytoin, chlorpromazine, interferon alpha, amoxicillin, and quinidine. APS frequently is associated with other systemic autoimmune disorders, most commonly SLE. Other common rheumatologic diseases associated with APS include Sjögren's syndrome, rheumatoid arthritis, autoimmune thrombocytopenic purpura, hemolytic anemia, psoriatic arthritis, systemic sclerosis, polymyalgia rheumatica, giant cell arteritis, and Behcet disease.

DIAGNOSTIC TOOLS
There are three aPL tests of clinical usefulness of determining the likelihood of thrombosis and assisting in the decision for treatment: LA as diluted Russell viper venom time (DRVVT), aCLs, and anti- β2GP1antibodies. Activated partial thromboplastin time (aPTT) may be an indicator for the presence of circulating LA. Work-up should include a complete blood count, a Coomb test, and serologic tests such as antinuclear antibody (ANA) and erythrocyte sedimentation rate (ESR). The aPL tests should be repeated on two occasions at least 12 weeks apart, as variability of the results may alter the course of

treatment. Neuroimaging studies with MRI of brain may show subcortical white matter changes, cerebral infarctions, or sinovenous occlusive disease [51,52].

Patients who have suspected VTE should undergo a Doppler sonography of the lower extremities, and when there is clinical suspicion, CT of the chest should be obtained to rule out pulmonary embolism. Echocardiogram should be performed in all patients who have APS presenting with strokes looking for cardiac thrombi or Libman Sacks endocarditis. Other causes of thromboembolic events should be excluded.

MANAGEMENT

Primary prevention is key in individuals who have persistently elevated aPL levels. Young women should avoid oral contraceptive use. Behavior risk factors modifications including smoking cessation and enhancing physical activity should be encouraged. Other modifiable vascular risk factors such as arterial hypertension, diabetes mellitus, and hyperlipidemia, should be controlled.

Primary Prevention

The optimal treatment for APS remains unclear in the absence of well-designed randomized clinical trials. Treatment should be focused on managing the underlying disorder. Prophylactic platelet antiaggregant therapy is not proven beneficial in asymptomatic individuals who have positive aPLs. As such, antigenecity carries a low absolute risk of thrombosis of less than 1% per year [53]. The Antiphospholipid Antibody Acetylsalicylic Acid (APLASA) study, a multicenter, randomized, double-blind, placebo-controlled clinical trial, showed no benefit for prophylactic antithrombotic therapy with low-dose aspirin in asymptomatic individuals who had circulating aPLs in the absence of prior thrombotic events [54].

Secondary Prevention

Although anticoagulants often are indicated in patients who have recurrent VTEs, the optimal duration and intensity of anticoagulation are disputable [55,56]. To date, there is not enough evidence to support the use of high-intensity warfarin (target international normalized ratio [INR] greater than 3.0) versus moderate-intensity warfarin in patients who have recurrent VTEs. The first randomized double-blind, controlled trial comparing two different doses of anticoagulation with warfarin for preventing recurrent thrombotic events in 114 patients with a mean follow up of 2.7 years showed that high-intensity anticoagulation (INR 3.1 to 4.0) was not superior to moderate-intensity anticoagulation (INR 2.0 to 3.0) [57]. Similarly, in a recent randomized trial of 109 patients who had APS followed for a mean of 3.9 years, high-intensity warfarin did not show superiority and was associated with an increased rate of minor hemorrhagic complications [56]. These studies suggest that standard anticoagulation therapy is sufficient for preventing recurrent VTEs in patients who have APS.

The best therapeutic strategy for preventing stroke in patients who have APS remains unclear. In patients who have stroke and APS, aspirin is as effective as moderate-intensity warfarin for preventing recurrent cerebral events. In a prospective cohort study of a subgroup of patients with ischemic stroke in the Warfarin-Aspirin Recurrent Stroke Study trial, aspirin 325 mg and warfarin (target INR 1.4 to 2.8) were equivalent for preventing recurrent strokes and VTEs over a 2-year follow up [26]. Low-dose aspirin carried a low risk of recurrent stroke of 3.5 per 100 patient-year in a small study of eight patients who had APS and first ischemic stroke during an 8.9-year follow-up [58]. Therefore, until further large prospective well-designed randomized clinical trials are available to determine best optimal treatment approach in patients who have APS and arterial cerebral infarctions, aspirin therapy may be sufficient as first-line therapy in primary APS with arterial ischemic stroke in the absence of venous thrombosis. Other antiplatelet agents shown to be beneficial in preventing atherosclerotic ischemic stroke, such as extended release dipyridamole in association with aspirin, or clopidogrel, may be used, but their efficacy in patients who have APS and ischemic stroke is not proven.

Antimalarial drugs such as chloroquine and hydroxychloroquine are disease-modifying agents useful in for preventing postoperative thrombosis and managing SLE and APS with or without SLE [59]. In recent experimental study, hydroxychloroquine inhibited platelet activation induced by aPLs [60]. Although their effect on prevention of further thrombosis has not been tested in prospective studies, antimalarial drugs may prove useful for treating APS.

In patients who have recurrent miscarriage associated with APS, treatment with heparin and low-dose aspirin may improve fetal survival as compared with aspirin alone [61–63]. Intravenous immune globulin therapy may reduce obstetric complications [64]. Because of its teratogenicity, warfarin should be avoided during pregnancy in APS and should be replaced by low molecular weight heparin (LMWH) or unfractionated heparin (UFH).

Catastrophic APS is a medical emergency and should be treated aggressively. Plasmapheresis and/or intravenous immunoglobulin therapy in combination with corticosteroids and anticoagulation may improve outcome [65–68]. The use of immunosuppressants such as cyclophosphamide, in combination with prednisone, may be beneficial, especially in patients who have underlying SLE. Newer treatments with rituximab have been described with variable response [69–71].

PROGNOSIS

Most patients continue to have recurrent thrombotic events despite aggressive therapies. An aCL level above 20 to 40 GPL among consecutive ischemic stroke patients is a marker of increased mortality during follow-up. Older age, higher rates of cardiovascular risk factors, and malignancy detected during follow-up account for the higher mortality [72]. The risk of recurrent thrombosis exceeds 10% per year in patients with prior history of venous thrombosis who have discontinued anticoagulant drugs within 6 months [53]. Fatal outcome may occur in patients who have recurrent myocardial infarctions, pulmonary embolism, and in more than half the patients who have catastrophic APS.

SUMMARY

The aPLs, specifically LA and anti-b2GP1 antibodies, increasingly are recognized as risk factors for stroke, especially in young adults. Positivity of aPLs in healthy individuals may not confer increased vascular thrombo–occlusive risk; therefore prophylactic use of antiaggregants in those individuals may not be necessary. Patients who have definite APS are at higher risk for recurrent VTEs, especially in the presence of SLE. The optimal treatment approach remains controversial. Long-term warfarin anticoagulation (INR 2.0 to 3.0) may be optimal in patients who have recurrent VTEs. Aspirin is acceptable for patients who have APS and first ischemic stroke in the absence of other underlying etiology for the ischemic event. Specific therapy and duration of treatment must be determined on an individual basis, taking into account the age, gender, severity of the event, recurrence, bleeding complications, and other risk factors for arterial of venous thromboembolism.

References

[1] Gharavi AE, Harris EN, Asherson RA, et al. Anticardiolipin antibodies: isotype distribution and phospholipid specificity. Ann Rheum Dis 1987;46(1):1–6.
[2] McNeil HP, Chesterman CN, Krilis SA. Anticardiolipin antibodies and lupus anticoagulants comprise separate antibody subgroups with different phospholipid binding characteristics. Br J Haematol 1989;73(4):506–13.
[3] Bevers EM, Galli M, Barbui T, et al. Lupus anticoagulant IgGs (LA) are not directed to phospholipids only, but to a complex of lipid-bound human prothrombin. Thromb Haemost 1991;66(6):629–32.
[4] Petri M. Epidemiology of the antiphospholipid antibody syndrome. J Autoimmun 2000;15(2):145–51.
[5] Love PE, Santoro SA. Antiphospholipid antibodies: anticardiolipin and the lupus anticoagulant in systemic lupus erythematosus (SLE) and in non-SLE disorders. Prevalence and clinical significance. Ann Intern Med 1990;112(9):682–98.
[6] Merkel PA, Chang Y, Pierangeli SS, et al. The prevalence and clinical associations of anticardiolipin antibodies in a large inception cohort of patients with connective tissue diseases. Am J Med 1996;101(6):576–83.
[7] Janardhan V, Wolf PA, Kase CS, et al. Anticardiolipin antibodies and risk of ischemic stroke and transient ischemic attack: the Framingham cohort and offspring study. Stroke 2004;35(3):736–41.
[8] Carreras LO, Forastiero RR, Martinuzzo ME. Which are the best biological markers of the antiphospholipid syndrome? J Autoimmun 2000;15(2):163–72.
[9] Galli M, Luciani D, Bertolini G, et al. Lupus anticoagulants are stronger risk factors for thrombosis than anticardiolipin antibodies in the antiphospholipid syndrome: a systematic review of the literature. Blood 2003;101(5):1827–32.
[10] Wilson WA, Gharavi AE, Koike T, et al. International consensus statement on preliminary classification criteria for definite antiphospholipid syndrome: report of an international workshop. Arthritis Rheum 1999;42(7):1309–11.
[11] Miyakis S, Lockshin MD, Atsumi T, et al. International consensus statement on an update of the classification criteria for definite antiphospholipid syndrome (APS). J Thromb Haemost 2006;4(2):295–306.

[12] Brey RL, Hart RG, Sherman DG, et al. Antiphospholipid antibodies and cerebral ischemia in young people. Neurology 1990;40(8):1190–6.
[13] Blohorn A, Guegan-Massardier E, Triquenot A, et al. Antiphospholipid antibodies in the acute phase of cerebral ischaemia in young adults: a descriptive study of 139 patients. Cerebrovasc Dis 2002;13(3):156–62.
[14] Singh K, Gaiha M, Shome DK, et al. The association of antiphospholipid antibodies with ischaemic stroke and myocardial infarction in young and their correlation: a preliminary study. J Assoc Physicians India 2001;49:527–9.
[15] Nagaraja D, Christopher R, Manjari T. Anticardiolipin antibodies in ischemic stroke in the young: Indian experience. J Neurol Sci 1997;150(2):137–42.
[16] Kushner MJ. Prospective study of anticardiolipin antibodies in stroke. Stroke 1990;21(2): 295–8.
[17] The Antiphospholipid Antibodies in Stroke Study (APASS) Group. Anticardiolipin antibodies are an independent risk factor for first ischemic stroke. Neurology 1993;43(10): 2069–73.
[18] Devilat M, Toso M, Morales M. Childhood stroke associated with protein C or S deficiency and primary antiphospholipid syndrome. Pediatr Neurol 1993;9(1):67–70.
[19] Tuhrim S, Rand JH, Wu XX, et al. Elevated anticardiolipin antibody titer is a stroke risk factor in a multiethnic population independent of isotype or degree of positivity. Stroke 1999;30(8):1561–5.
[20] Tuhrim S, Rand JH, Wu X, et al. Antiphosphatidyl serine antibodies are independently associated with ischemic stroke. Neurology 1999;53(7):1523–7.
[21] Zielinska J, Ryglewicz D, Wierzchowska E, et al. Anticardiolipin antibodies are an independent risk factor for ischemic stroke. Neurol Res 1999;21(7):653–7.
[22] Toschi V, Motta A, Castelli C, et al. High prevalence of antiphosphatidylinositol antibodies in young patients with cerebral ischemia of undetermined cause. Stroke 1998;29(9): 1759–64.
[23] Levine SR, Brey RL, Joseph CL, et al. Risk of recurrent thromboembolic events in patients with focal cerebral ischemia and antiphospholipid antibodies. The Antiphospholipid Antibodies in Stroke Study Group. Stroke 1992;23(2 Suppl):I29–32.
[24] Brey RL, Abbott RD, Curb JD, et al. beta(2)-Glycoprotein 1-dependent anticardiolipin antibodies and risk of ischemic stroke and myocardial infarction: the Honolulu heart program. Stroke 2001;32(8):1701–6.
[25] Brey RL, Stallworth CL, McGlasson DL, et al. Antiphospholipid antibodies and stroke in young women. Stroke 2002;33(10):2396–400.
[26] Levine SR, Brey RL, Tilley BC, et al. Antiphospholipid antibodies and subsequent thrombo-occlusive events in patients with ischemic stroke. JAMA 2004;291(5):576–84.
[27] Fustinoni O, Biller J. Recurrent cerebral infarcts in antiphospholipid syndrome. In: Rabinstein AA, Wijdicks EFM, editors. Tough calls in acute neurology. Philadelphia: Elsevier; 2004. p. 199–215.
[28] Milstone A, Fan A, Fuchs H. Antiphospholipid syndrome associated with seizures. South Med J 1996;89(7):738–40.
[29] Manna R, Ricci V, Curigliano V, et al. Psychiatric manifestations as a primary symptom in antiphospholipid syndrome. Int J Immunopathol Pharmacol 2006;19(4):915–7.
[30] Gomez-Puerta JA, Cervera R, Calvo LM, et al. Dementia associated with the antiphospholipid syndrome: clinical and radiological characteristics of 30 patients. Rheumatology (Oxford) 2005;44(1):95–9.
[31] Rafai MA, Fadel H, Gam I, et al. [Recurrent stroke revealing catastrophic antiphospholipid syndrome with hepatitis C viral infection]. Rev Neurol (Paris) 2006;162(11):1131–4 [in French].
[32] Carter D, Olchovsky D, Yonath H, et al. Simultaneous deep vein thrombosis and transverse myelitis with negative serology as a first sign of antiphospholipid syndrome: a case report and review of the literature. Clin Rheumatol 2006;25(5):756–8.

[33] Besbas N, Anlar B, Apak A, et al. Optic neuropathy in primary antiphospholipid syndrome in childhood. J Child Neurol 2001;16(9):690–3.
[34] Ijdo JW, Conti-Kelly AM, Greco P, et al. Antiphospholipid antibodies in patients with multiple sclerosis and MS-like illnesses: MS or APS? Lupus 1999;8(2):109–15.
[35] Garg N, Zivadinov R, Ramanathan M, et al. Clinical and MRI correlates of autoreactive antibodies in multiple sclerosis patients. J Neuroimmunol 2007;187:159–65.
[36] Avcin T, Markelj G, Niksic V, et al. Estimation of antiphospholipid antibodies in a prospective longitudinal study of children with migraine. Cephalalgia 2004;24(10):831–7.
[37] Tietjen GE. Migraine and antiphospholipid antibodies. Cephalalgia 1992;12(2):69–74.
[38] Nakos G, Tziakou E, Maneta-Peyret L, et al. Antiphospholipid antibodies in serum from patients with Guillain-Barre syndrome. Intensive Care Med 2005;31(10):1401–8.
[39] Cavallasca JA, Gutierrez DM, Bercellini EA, et al. Sudden sensorineural hearing loss as a manifestation of primary antiphospholipid syndrome. Joint Bone Spine 2007;74:403–4.
[40] Kang KT, Young YH. Sudden sensorineural hearing loss in a patient with primary antiphospholipid syndrome. J Laryngol Otol 2007;1–3.
[41] Wiles NM, Hunt BJ, Callanan V, et al. Sudden sensorineural hearing loss and antiphospholipid syndrome. Haematologica 2006;91:e124–7.
[42] Chapman J, Rand JH, Brey RL, et al. Nonstroke neurological syndromes associated with antiphospholipid antibodies: evaluation of clinical and experimental studies. Lupus 2003;12(7):514–7.
[43] Martino D, Chew NK, Mir P, et al. Atypical movement disorders in antiphospholipid syndrome. Mov Disord 2006;21(7):944–9.
[44] Frances C, Niang S, Laffitte E, et al. Dermatologic manifestations of the antiphospholipid syndrome: two hundred consecutive cases. Arthritis Rheum 2005;52(6):1785–93.
[45] Turiel M, Sarzi-Puttini P, Peretti R, et al. Five-year follow-up by transesophageal echocardiographic studies in primary antiphospholipid syndrome. Am J Cardiol 2005;96(4):574–9.
[46] Asherson RA. Multiorgan failure and antiphospholipid antibodies: the catastrophic antiphospholipid (Asherson's) syndrome. Immunobiology 2005;210(10):727–33.
[47] Miesbach W, Asherson RA, Cervera R, et al. The catastrophic antiphospholipid (Asherson's) syndrome and malignancies. Autoimmun Rev 2006;6(2):94–7.
[48] Bucciarelli S, Espinosa G, Cervera R, et al. Mortality in the catastrophic antiphospholipid syndrome: causes of death and prognostic factors in a series of 250 patients. Arthritis Rheum 2006;54(8):2568–76.
[49] Bucciarelli S, Cervera R, Espinosa G, et al. Mortality in the catastrophic antiphospholipid syndrome: causes of death and prognostic factors. Autoimmun Rev 2006;6(2):72–5.
[50] Bayraktar UD, Erkan D, Bucciarelli S, et al. The clinical spectrum of catastrophic antiphospholipid syndrome in the absence and presence of lupus. J Rheumatol 2007;34(2):346–52.
[51] Csepany T, Bereczki D, Kollar J, et al. MRI findings in central nervous system systemic lupus erythematosus are associated with immunoserological parameters and hypertension. J Neurol 2003;250(11):1348–54.
[52] Provenzale JM, Heinz ER, Ortel TL, et al. Antiphospholipid antibodies in patients without systemic lupus erythematosus: neuroradiologic findings. Radiology 1994;192(2):531–7.
[53] Lim W, Crowther MA, Eikelboom JW. Management of antiphospholipid antibody syndrome: a systematic review. JAMA 2006;295(9):1050–7.
[54] Erkan D, Harrison MJ, Levy R, et al. Aspirin for primary thrombosis prevention in the antiphospholipid syndrome: a randomized, double-blind, placebo-controlled trial in asymptomatic antiphospholipid antibody-positive individuals. Arthritis Rheum 2007;56(7):2382–91.
[55] Khamashta MA, Cuadrado MJ, Mujic F, et al. The management of thrombosis in the antiphospholipid–antibody syndrome. N Engl J Med 1995;332(15):993–7.
[56] Finazzi G, Marchioli R, Brancaccio V, et al. A randomized clinical trial of high-intensity warfarin vs. conventional antithrombotic therapy for the prevention of recurrent thrombosis in patients with the antiphospholipid syndrome (WAPS). J Thromb Haemost 2005;3(5):848–53.

[57] Crowther MA, Ginsberg JS, Julian J, et al. A comparison of two intensities of warfarin for the prevention of recurrent thrombosis in patients with the antiphospholipid antibody syndrome. N Engl J Med 2003;349(12):1133–8.
[58] Derksen RH, de Groot PG, Kappelle LJ. Low dose aspirin after ischemic stroke associated with antiphospholipid syndrome. Neurology 2003;61(1):111–4.
[59] Wallace DJ. Antimalarial agents and lupus. Rheum Dis Clin North Am 1994;20(1): 243–63.
[60] Espinola RG, Pierangeli SS, Gharavi AE, et al. Hydroxychloroquine reverses platelet activation induced by human IgG antiphospholipid antibodies. Thromb Haemost 2002;87(3): 518–22.
[61] Rai R, Cohen H, Dave M, et al. Randomised controlled trial of aspirin and aspirin plus heparin in pregnant women with recurrent miscarriage associated with phospholipid antibodies (or antiphospholipid antibodies). BMJ 1997;314(7076):253–7.
[62] Girardi G, Redecha P, Salmon JE. Heparin prevents antiphospholipid antibody-induced fetal loss by inhibiting complement activation. Nat Med 2004;10(11):1222–6.
[63] Glasnovic M, Bosnjak I, Vcev A, et al. Antibody profile of pregnant women with antiphospholipid syndrome and pregnancy outcome after treatment with low-dose aspirin and low-weight molecular heparin. Coll Antropol 2007;31(1):173–7.
[64] Branch DW, Peaceman AM, Druzin M, et al. A multicenter, placebo-controlled pilot study of intravenous immune globulin treatment of antiphospholipid syndrome during pregnancy. The Pregnancy Loss Study Group. Am J Obstet Gynecol 2000;182(1 Pt 1):122–7.
[65] Ruffatti A, Marson P, Pengo V, et al. Plasma exchange in the management of high-risk pregnant patients with primary antiphospholipid syndrome. A report of 9 cases and a review of the literature. Autoimmun Rev 2007;6(3):196–202.
[66] Uthman I, Shamseddine A, Taher A. The role of therapeutic plasma exchange in the catastrophic antiphospholipid syndrome. Transfus Apher Sci 2005;33(1):11–7.
[67] Erkan D. Therapeutic and prognostic considerations in catastrophic antiphospholipid syndrome. Autoimmun Rev 2006;6(2):98–103.
[68] Cervera R, Asherson RA, Font J. Catastrophic antiphospholipid syndrome. Rheum Dis Clin North Am 2006;32(3):575–90.
[69] Rubenstein E, Arkfeld DG, Metyas S, et al. Rituximab treatment for resistant antiphospholipid syndrome. J Rheumatol 2006;33(2):355–7.
[70] Trappe R, Loew A, Thuss-Patience P, et al. Successful treatment of thrombocytopenia in primary antiphospholipid antibody syndrome with the anti-CD20 antibody rituximab—monitoring of antiphospholipid and anti-GP antibodies: a case report. Ann Hematol 2006;85(2):134–5.
[71] Merrill JT. Rituximab in antiphospholipid syndrome. Curr Rheumatol Rep 2003;5(5):381–2.
[72] Tanne D, D'Olhaberriague L, Trivedi AM, et al. Anticardiolipin antibodies and mortality in patients with ischemic stroke: a prospective follow-up study. Neuroepidemiology 2002;21(2):93–9.

Antiphospholipid Syndrome in Pregnancy

Rodger L. Bick, MD, PhD, FACP

10455 North Central Expressway, Suite 109-320, Dallas, TX 75231, USA

Antiphospholipid syndrome (APLS) causes significant difficulties in obstetrics and pregnancy, including maternal thrombosis, fetal growth retardation, infertility, and recurrent miscarriage syndrome (RMS). The most common of these, by far, is RMS. RMS is a common obstetric problem, affecting more than 500,000 women in the United States each year [1]. Infertility, although less well defined in the population, also is a common clinical problem.

Recurrent miscarriage, based on literature available and the authors' experience, generally is caused by well-defined defects. About 7% of cases are secondary to chromosomal abnormalities, about 10% are caused by anatomic abnormalities, about 15% seem to be caused by hormonal abnormalities (progesterone, estrogens, diabetes, or thyroid disease), about 6% cannot be explained, and the remainder, about 55% to 62%, are caused by blood coagulation protein/platelet defects [1]. The most common cause of RMS, however, is APLS.

RECURRENT MISCARRIAGE SYNDROME AND ANTIPHOSPHOLIPID SYNDROME

The thrombotic defect of APLS associated with fetal wastage is thought to be caused by thrombosis of early placental vessels. Fetal wastage peaks in the first trimester, but small peaks also occur in the second and third trimesters [1,2]. It seems that the earlier the pregnancy, the smaller are the placental and uterine vessels, and therefore the greater is the vessels' propensity to undergo partial or total occlusion by thrombus formation. Thrombotic occlusion of placental vessels, both venous and arterial, precludes adequate nutrition and thus affects the viability of the fetus [1,2].

The defects in thrombotic hemostasis associated with RMS include lupus anticoagulants, anticardiolipin antibodies, and subgroup antiphospholipid antibodies (all of these comprise APLS associated with fetal wastage syndrome) [3–5].

Of all hereditary and acquired procoagulant defects (thrombophilias), APLS is clearly the most common thrombotic defect leading to fetal wastage

E-mail address: rbick@thromosis.com

syndrome/infertility, and a variety of treatment programs have been advocated. One difficulty in evaluating these programs has been that some studies primarily addressed patients who had secondary APLS and fetal wastage, in particular patients who had underlying systemic lupus erythematosus or other autoimmune disorders. Only a few investigators have addressed populations of patients who had primary APLS, with no known underlying disease.

APLS has long been recognized as a cause of miscarriage and infertility; it also has long been recognized that treatment is often successful [6]. Many clinicians consider APLS to be the most common prothrombotic disorder among both hereditary and acquired defects and the most common thrombotic disorder causing recurrent miscarriage [1,2,7–11]. When assessing causes of infertility alone, APLS is thought to account for about 30% of infertility. In one series, however, abnormal CD56+/CD16 cell ratios were the single most common defect found in infertility patients (40%) [12]. In another recent series, only 21% of patients who had RMS had APLS; however, an historical assessment of assessing women who had APLS found that 80% had suffered at least one miscarriage [13]. In a series reported by Granger [14], 384 unselected patients were assessed for APLS. Of these, 16% harbored APLS, and 56% of those who had APLS were treated with low-dose aspirin and had a term delivery [14]. Borelli [15] found that 60% of patients who had "habitual" unexplained miscarriage harbored APLS. Although most cases of APLS are clearly acquired [9,10], familial APLS associated with RMS has been reported [16]. Clearly, however, screening for APLS is indicated in patients who have RMS [1–4,7,8,10,17]. One recent study has suggested that using prothrombin fragment 1.2 to monitor patients who have APLS and have experienced miscarriage may predict preclinical placental thrombi [18]. If this finding is confirmed, it may preclude the need for frequent sonograms, which is the current mode of careful following pregnant patients who are receiving therapy for RMS . In addition, because APLS is so common and because many of the hereditary thrombophilias, such as factor V Leiden, are so prevalent in North America, it is to be expected that some women who have RMS harbor APLS in combination with other procoagulant defects. Aznar [19] has reported a case of RMS complicated by deep vein thrombosis and thrombotic stroke in a patient who had APLS, factor V Leiden, and congenital protein S deficiency [19]. Many mechanisms whereby APLS interferes with the hemostasis system and predisposes patients to thrombosis have been proposed [1–4,7–10,17]. Some investigators, however, have proposed mechanisms specific for RMS. These suggested mechanisms have included the proposal the APLS induces acquired activated protein C resistance [20] and/or interferes with prothrombin (factor II), protein C and protein S, tissue factor, factor XI [21], and the tissue factor/tissue factor pathway inhibitor system [22]. Another study also found that patients who had APLS also harbored antibodies to prothrombin, protein C, and protein S [23]. Others have proposed these patients also may develop antibodies to thromboplastin and thrombin [24]. Another proposal is that antiphospholipid antibodies interfere with annexin-V (also known as "placental anticoagulant protein") [25]. Two studies have shown that immunoglobulin fractions of antiphospholipid antibody or beta-2-glycoprotein-1 decrease trophoblastic annexin-V [25–27], but several others have shown this anti-annexin-V activity to be limited to the anti-phosphatidlyserine subgroup antibody idiotype [28,29]. Two carefully done studies failed to demonstrate abnormalities of annexin-V in patients who had APLS and experienced miscarriage. These investigators concluded that annexin-V plays no role in RMS [30,31]. In an additional study, anti-annexin antibodies were detected in only 19% of patients who had lupus; however, these patients had not suffered miscarriage [32]. In an additional study in patients who had lupus but who did not have RMS, only 3.8% harbored anti-annexin-V antibodies [21]. In yet another study that assessed patients who had thrombosis and APLS, only 8% harbored beta-2-glycoprotein-1 [33]. Testing for an antiphospholipid subgroup, in this case anti-phosphatidylserine, was found useful in one study in which patients who had RMS were negative for lupus anticoagulants and anticardiolipin antibodies [34]. In another study, however, the use of APL subgroup testing was not considered helpful [35]. It should be noted that on rare occasions APLS may be inherited (this author has seen three such families, and other cases have been reported) [16]. This experience suggests that a positive maternal history may warrant evaluation at first pregnancy, as should a history of familial thrombosis.

Patients harboring other congenital or acquired thrombophilic states are also at high risk for placental thrombosis and RMS. In one study assessing a variety of these defects in 46 selected women who had RMS (anatomic and hormonal defects were ruled out before hemostasis assessment), 76% had anticardiolipin antibodies (void of lupus anticoagulants), 3% had a lupus anticoagulant (void of anticardiolipin antibodies), 11% had congenital protein S deficiency (three quantitative and one dysfunctional), 6.5% had sticky platelet syndrome (two had type I, and one had type II), 3% had dysfibrinogenemia, and 3% had congenital tissue plasminogen activator (tPA) deficiency [36].

The antiphospholipid antibodies that are important in pregnancy and obstetrics are listed in Box 1. The potential and proposed mechanism(s) of antiphospholipid antibody – induced thrombosis in pregnancy are summarized in Box 2.

ANTIPHOSPHOLIPID ANTIBODIES VERSUS OTHER THROMBOPHILIAS LEADING TO RECURRENT MISCARRIAGE SYNDROME: THE DALLAS THROMBOSIS HEMOSTASIS CLINICAL CENTER EXPERIENCE

During the past 5 years the author and colleagues at the Dallas Thrombosis Hemostasis Clinical Center have carefully assessed 351 women referred for evaluation of thrombosis and hemostasis after they had suffered recurrent miscarriages. In the Dallas/Fort Worth Metroplex (DFW Metroplex), with a population of about 6 million, a flow protocol is followed to maximize success and keep the costs of evaluation of RMS/infertility at a minimum while providing the best chances for defining a cause and thus providing optimal therapy for successful term pregnancy outcome [1,2,36]. This protocol is presented in

> **Box 1: Important antiphospholipid antibodies that are important in recurrent miscarriage syndrome**
>
> Anticardiolipin antibodies (IgG, IgA, IgM)
> Beta-2-glycoprotein-1 (IgG, IgA, IgM)
> Anti-phosphatidylserine (IgG, IgA, IgM)
> Anti-phosphatidylinositol (IgG, IgA, IgM)
> Anti-phosphatidylcholine (IgG, IgA, IgM)
> Anti-phosphatidic acid (IgG, IgA, IgM)
> Anti-phosphatidylethanolamine (IgG, IgA, IgM)
> Anti-phosphatidic acid (IgG, IgA, IgM)
> Anti-phosphatidylglycerol (IgG, IgA, IgM)
> Anti-annexin-v antibody (IgG, IgA, IgM)
> Lupus anticoagulant
> Hexagonal phospholipid

Fig. 1. In all instances, women who have RMS/infertility are seen first by an obstetrician or reproductive specialist. At this stage anatomic defects and hormonal defects are assessed. If such defects are found (as happens in about 24% of the women seen), the work-up ends, and treatment is initiated. If no anatomic or hormonal defect is found, the patient is referred for hemostasis evaluation; the positive yield among this selected population is about 92%. If this evaluation is negative (in about 8% of women referred), chromosomal evaluation (with a yield of about 7%) is initiated if the patient desires. Most of the obstetricians/reproductive specialists in the DFW Metroplex refer patients for work-up after two or more miscarriages; however, some refer after one

> **Box 2: Proposed mechanisms of thrombosis of antiphospholipid antibodies**
>
> 1. Interference with endothelial phospholipids and thus prostacyclin release
> 2. Inhibition of prekallikrein and thus inhibition of fibrinolysis
> 3. Inhibition of thrombomodulin and thus protein C/S activity
> 4. Acquired protein C resistance (nonmolecular)
> 5. Interaction with platelet membrane phospholipids
> 6. Inhibition of endothelial tPA release
> 7. Direct inhibition of protein S
> 8. Inhibition of annexin-V, a cell surface protein that inhibits tissue factor, also referred to as "placental anticoagulant protein" (serine only)
> 9. Induction of the release of monocyte tissue factor

ANTIPHOSPHOLIPID SYNDROME IN PREGNANCY

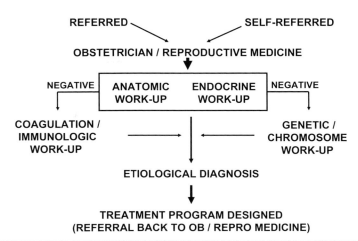

Fig. 1. Dallas Ft. Worth Metroplex algorithm for work-up of a woman who has recurrent miscarriage syndrome.

miscarriage in the face of a positive family history for miscarriage. Occasionally, patients request a work-up after only one miscarriage. The practice of the authors and colleagues has been to accommodate the desires of the patient, after discussing the costs and other implications of evaluation. At the time of this writing, all 322 patients who had a defect have been followed for at least 15 months and thus have been analyzed in detail, as presented in the following section.

CHARACTERISTICS OF THE FIRST 351 WOMEN REFERRED FOR HEMOSTASIS EVALUATION

The mean age of patients referred for a hemostasis evaluation was 33.3 years, the mean number of miscarriages before referral was 2.9 (range, 2–9), and the percentage found to have a hemostasis defect was 92% (Table 1).

All patients underwent a thorough evaluation for thrombophilia and, when indicated, for a hemorrhagic disorder. Of the 351 patients, 29 (8%) had no defect. Of the remaining 322 patients, 7 (2%) had a bleeding disorder: three

Table 1
The Dallas Thrombosis Hemostasis Clinical Center experience: patient demographics

Patient characteristics (n = 351)	Mean	SD	Maximum	Minimum
Age	33.3	5.63	49	18
Number of miscarriages:	2.9	2.39	9	2
Percentage with defects (322/351)	92			

had platelet dysfunction, one had factor XIII deficiency, three had von Willebrand's factor, and three had Osler-Weber-Rendu syndrome. The remainder of the patients had a thrombophilia: the great majority (195, 60%) had antiphospholipid syndrome; 64 (20%) had sticky platelet syndrome; 38 (12%) had methylene tetrahydrofolate reductase (MTHFR) mutation; 23 (7.1%) had plasminogen activator inhibitor 1 (PAI-1) polymorphism; 12 (3.7%) had protein S deficiency; 12 (3.7%) had factor V Leiden, 3 (1%); had antithrombin (AT) deficiency; 3 (1%) had heparin-cofactor II deficiency; 3 (1%) had tPA deficiency; and 6 (2%) had protein C deficiency. A total of 364 defects were found in the 312 patients harboring thrombophilia; thus, several patients harbored two defects, and a few harbored three separate defects.

Similar to reports by most other investigators, as discussed previously, the most common defect found was APLS. Unlike some groups, however, the author and colleagues assess for all phospholipid antibody subgroups including anti-phosphatidylserine, anti-phosphatidylethanolamine, anti-phosphatidylglycerol, anti-phosphatidic acid, anti-phosphatidylcholine, anti-phosphatidylinositol, anti-annexin-V antibody, beta-2-glycoprotein-1, hexagonal phospholipid, and lupus anticoagulant (by dilute Russell's viper venom time) with correction by non–platelet-derived phospholipid to avoid false-positive results). They always assess all three idiotypes of anticardiolipin antibody (IgG, IgA and IgM); many who evaluate such patients continue to make an incomplete evaluation, leaving out either IgA or IgM idiotypes. The defects identified by the author's group, in order of frequency, are summarized in Box 3. When all antiphospholipid subgroups are included, 29% of patients are found to have a subgroup antiphospholipid antibody but no anticardiolipin antibody or lupus anticoagulant; thus 29% of patients would remain undiagnosed if assays for these subgroups were not performed. This finding is about equivalent to the finding recently noted in young (< 51 years) patients who had had thrombotic stroke [37]. The hemostasis defects found in the author's population are summarized in Box 3. The particulars of the patients who had antiphospholipid antibodies, with demonstration of the idiotypes found, are summarized in Table 2.

All patients who had a thrombophilic defect, including APLS, were treated with preconception aspirin at 81 mg/d. At documentation of conception, the first 120 patients were treated with the addition of subcutaneous self-injected unfractionated porcine mucosal heparin at 5000 units every 12 hours. The subsequent 192 patients were treated with subcutaneous self-injected low molecular weight (LMW) heparin dalteparin (Fragmin) at 5000 units every 24 hours by self-injection. Both drugs (aspirin plus unfractionated heparin or LMW heparin) are used to term. All patients are instructed in injecting heparin and are informed extensively of the benefits and risks of heparin/LMW heparin therapy, including side effects that, although rare, can include heparin-induced thrombocytopenia (HIT) with and without paradoxical thrombosis/thromboembolism (HITT); osteoporosis; mild to moderate alopecia; skin and allergic reactions, including erythema and itching, at injection sites; eosinophilia (of

> **Box 3: Hemostasis defects found in patients who had suffered recurrent miscarriage**[a]
>
> *Thrombotic defects*
> Antiphospholipid syndrome: 195 (60%)
> Sticky platelet syndrome: 64 (20%)
> MTHFR mutation: 38 (12%)
> Pai-1 polymorphism: 12 (3.7%)
> Protein s deficiency: 12 (3.7%)
> Factor V Leiden: 12 (3.7%)
> Antithrombin deficiency: 3 (1%)
> Heparin cofactor II deficiency: 3 (1%)
> tPA deficiency: 3 (1%)
> Protein C deficiency: 6 (2%)
>
> *Hemorrhagic defects*
> Platelet dysfunction: 3
> Factor XIII deficiency: 1
> Von Willebrand's disease: 3
> Osler-Weber-Rendu: 3
>
> [a]Some patients had two or three defects.

little clinical consequence); and potential bleeding. Patients also are informed that about 5% to 10% of patients develop a transient transaminasemia during heparin/LMW heparin therapy, but this transaminasemia is without any known adverse clinical consequences. They also are instructed that the ideal injection sites are the anterior or lateral thighs; that injection sites should be rotated with every injection; that each injection is likely to produce a bruise about 0.5 cm to 4.0 cm in diameter; and that pain of injection, if experienced, usually can be alleviated by applying a small piece of ice at the site for 20 seconds before and 20 seconds after the injection is given. All patients are instructed to return immediately if they note dark or black areas at the injection site, potentially indicative of skin necrosis. The methods of follow-up are summarized in Box 4.

Clinicians considering the use of one of the US Food and Drug Administration (FDA)-approved LMW heparins in pregnancy should be aware of the Medwatch Alert posted by the FDA in January 2002 regarding the use of enoxaparin (Lovenox) in pregnancy and women of childbearing age (Box 5) [38].

OUTCOMES

All of the 315 patients who had a thrombophilic defect were treated with the regimen of preconception low-dose aspirin plus postconception

Table 2
Antiphospholipids found in patients who have antiphospholipid syndrome (APLS)

Antiphospholipid identified	Percentage of patients who have APLS
ACLA-IgG only	32.6
ACLA-IgM only	23.4
ACLA-IgA only	7
ACLA-IgG + IgM	3
ACLA-IgG + IgA	1
ACLA IgA + IgM	0
Lupus anticoagulant only	2
ACLA + lupus anticoagulant	2
Subgroup only[a]	
Anti-phosphatidylserine	4
Anti-phosphatidylinositol	2
Anti-phosphatidylethanolamine	5
Anti-phosphatidic acid	5
Anti-phosphatidylcholine	7
Anti-phosphatidylglycerol	1
Anti-annexin-V	5
Beta-2-glycoprotein 1	0
Hexagonal phospholipid	0
Patients who had APLS and only a subgroup antibody (n = 9):	29

Abbreviation: ACLA, anticardiolipin antibody.
[a] No ACLA or LA present.

thromboprophylactic (low-dose) subcutaneous porcine heparin or thromboprophylactic doses of dalteparin. There were four losses (2.6%), only two of which were treatment failures. A loss during the second trimester that accompanied a cholecystectomy and a loss during the first trimester of a fetus that had a chromosomal defect in a woman who had APLS were not considered treatment (aspirin plus heparin/LMW heparin) failures. In two first-trimester losses in patients receiving aspirin plus heparin/LMW heparin, however, placental thrombi and infarcts were present; thus these two losses clearly represented treatment failure. The program's overall success in treating patients who had RMS with thrombophilic defects therefore was 99% (312/315) with respect to normal-term delivery. All patients were followed for a minimum of 3 months after delivery. No patient sustained a thrombotic episode during pregnancy, delivery, or postpartum, except the two treatment failures, both of whom had placental vascular thrombi. In addition, no patient developed HIT/HITT, and none had a clinically significant hemorrhage. Almost all patients developed small ecchymoses at injection sites, but these were considered insignificant by both patient and physician. Ten percent of patients developed eosinophilia that abated by 3 months postpartum, and 7% developed mild to moderate elevations of hepatic transaminases; these levels also returned to normal by 3 months postpartum. Reports from obstetricians, reproductive

> **Box 4: Protocol for recurrent miscarriage syndrome associated with antiphospholipid syndrome and other hypercoagulable defects (follow-up used by the DFW Metroplex Cooperative RMS Group)**
>
> *Medications: all are taken throughout pregnancy*
> 1. Aspirin, 81 mg/d, started preconception (at time of diagnosis)
> 2. Porcine heparin, 5000 units subcutaneously every 12 hours immediately postconception (added to aspirin; both taken to term) or dalteparin, 5000 units subcutaneously every 24 hours immediately postconception (added to aspirin and both taken to term)
> 3. Calcium, 500 mg/d, by mouth
> 4. Prenatal vitamins
> 5. Iron, 1 tablet per day, by mouth
> 6. Folic acid, 1 mg/d, by mouth
>
> *Laboratory assessment*
> 1. Complete blood cell (CBC)/platelet count and heparin level[a] weekly for 4 weeks, then
> 2. CBC/platelet count and heparin level monthly, to term
> 3. Sonogram initially, and frequently to term
> 4. Fetal activity charted daily starting at 28 weeks
> 5. Biophysical profile and color Doppler flow of umbilical artery at 32, 34, 36, and 38 weeks
> 6. Delivery at the discretion of the obstetrician
> 7. At delivery (or loss), send placenta to pathology for analysis and search for placental vascular thrombosis
>
> [a]By anti-Xa method.

medicine specialists, and involved pediatricians indicate that no neonatal or pediatric problems were associated with therapy. No patient sustained a fracture during or after treatment.

TREATMENT REVIEW

The author and his colleagues do not advocate using corticosteroid therapy in this population that has APLS, based on the negative experience of others in fetal wastage syndrome and their own preliminary experience of using steroids, in conjunction with antithrombotics, in patients who had APLS. They found that corticosteroid use lowered antiphospholipid antibody titers but failed to abort thrombotic events [1]. In addition, it is thought that steroid use may be detrimental in patients who have APLS [6].

A variety of treatment programs have been used for women who have antiphospholipids (anticardiolipin antibodies or lupus anticoagulants) and fetal

Box 5: [January 9, 2002: Aventis]

Warnings

Prosthetic Heart Valves: The use of Lovenox Injection is not recommended for thromboprophylaxis in patients with prosthetic heart valves. Cases of prosthetic heart valve thrombosis have been reported in patients with prosthetic valves who have received enoxaparin for thromboprophylaxis. Some of these cases were pregnant women in whom thrombosis led to maternal deaths and fetal deaths. Pregnant women with prosthetic heart valves may be at higher risk for thromboembolism (see Precautions: Pregnancy).

Precautions

Pregnancy

Teratogenic Effects

Second paragraph added:

> There have been reports of congenital anomalies in infants born to women who received enoxaparin during pregnancy including cerebral anomalies, limb anomalies, hypospadias, peripheral vascular malformation, fibrotic dysplasia, and cardiac defect. A cause and effect relationship has not been established nor has the incidence been shown to be higher than in the general population.

Non-Teratogenic Effects

First paragraph revised:

> There have been post-marketing reports of fetal death when pregnant women received Lovenox Injection. Causality for these cases has not been determined. Pregnant women receiving anti-coagulants, including enoxaparin, are at increased risk for bleeding. Hemorrhage can occur at any site and may lead to death of mother and/or fetus. Pregnant women receiving enoxaparin should be carefully monitored. Pregnant women and women of childbearing potential should be apprised of the potential hazard to the fetus and the mother if enoxaparin is administered during pregnancy.

Second paragraph added:

> In a clinical study of pregnant women with prosthetic heart valves given enoxaparin (1 mg/kg bid) to reduce the risk of thromboembolism, 2 of 7 women developed clots resulting in blockage of the valve and leading to maternal and fetal death. There are postmarketing reports of prosthetic valve thrombosis in pregnant women with prosthetic heart valves while receiving enoxaparin for thromboprophylaxis. These events resulted in maternal death or surgical interventions. The use of Lovenox Injection is not recommended for thromboprophylaxis in pregnant women with prosthetic heart valves (see WARNINGS: Prosthetic Heart Valves).

Adverse reactions

Ongoing Safety Surveillance: Since 1993, there have been over 80 reports of epidural or spinal hematoma formation with concurrent use of Lovenox Injection and spinal/epidural anesthesia or spinal puncture.

wastage syndrome; however, many of these studies have studied only very small populations or fail to distinguish between primary or secondary APLS in the information provided. Brown [39] reported a 90% failure rate (miscarriage) among untreated women, Perino [40] reports a 93% failure rate in untreated women, and Many [41] reports a 93% failure rate in untreated patients. Lubbe [42], noted a successful term pregnancy rate of 80% with use of prednisone and aspirin in a small group of women, and Lin [43] noted a similar success rate with this regimen. Cowchuck [44] noted a 75% success rate with prednisone alone or aspirin alone but also noted more undesirable effects in the prednisone-treated population. Landy [45], in a small population, reported a success rate of 90% with either aspirin alone or prednisone alone. Many [41], however, noted only a 43% successful term pregnancy rate with aspirin and prednisone, and Semprini [46] noted only a 14% success rate with prednisone alone. Several studies have assessed the postconception addition of heparin, but most have used higher doses than were used in the population treated by the author and colleagues. Rosove [47] reports a 93% success rate with dose-adjusted subcutaneous heparin, the mean heparin doses being about 25,000 units/d. Kutteh and Ermel [48], in a population of 25 patients treated with aspirin plus dose-adjusted subcutaneous heparin, noted a success rate of 76%; the mean heparin dose was 26,000 units/d. In Many's study [41], patients treated with prednisone plus aspirin plus heparin (5000 units twice a day) had a better outcome (69%) than did those treated with aspirin plus prednisone (43%) or prednisone alone (7%). Based on the author and colleagues' original and current results [1,2,36], fixed low-dose porcine heparin seems to be more effective than the high-dose, dose-adjusted regimens, with a normal term delivery by more than 98% of the RMS population that had APLS or other prothrombotic propensity. It may be that higher doses of heparin somehow contribute to adverse outcomes, such as small periplacental hemorrhages. Parke [49] reports on the combination of low-dose heparin used in conjunction with intravenous immunoglobulin. Her success rate, however, was only 27%, suggesting that intravenous immunoglobulin has little role in antiphospholipid fetal wastage syndrome.

SUMMARY

RMS and infertility are common problems in the United States with recurrent miscarriage effecting more than 500,000 women annually. If these women are properly screened through a cost-effective protocol, as outlined in this article, and a thorough APLS evaluation is performed, the most common thrombophilic defect found is APLS. Other hereditary and acquired procoagulant defects are also commonly found if looked for. It is important to evaluate women who have RMS appropriately, because, if a cause is found, most will have positive outcomes with normal term delivery. Treatment of the common procoagulant defects consists of preconception low-dose aspirin at 81 mg/d followed by the addition of low-dose unfractionated porcine heparin or dalteparin immediately after conception. Based on the author and colleagues' experience, LMH heparin may be a suitable alternative.

References

[1] Bick RL. Recurrent miscarriage syndrome and infertility caused by blood coagulation/platelet defects. In: Bick RL, Frenkel EP, Baker WF, et al, editors. Hematological complications of obstetrics, pregnancy and gynecology. Cambridge (UK): Cambridge University Press; 2006. p. 55–74.
[2] Bick RL. Recurrent miscarriage syndrome and infertility caused by blood coagulation protein or platelet defects. Hematol Oncol Clin North Am 2000;14:1117–32.
[3] Bick RL, Baker WF. Antiphospholipid syndrome and thrombosis. Semin Thromb Hemost 1999;25:333–50.
[4] Bick RL. The antiphospholipid thrombosis syndromes: a common multidisciplinary medical problem. Clin Appl Thromb Hemost 1997;3:270–83.
[5] Scott JR, Rote NS, Branch DW. Immunological aspects of recurrent abortion and fetal death. Obstet Gynecol 1987;70:645–56.
[6] Khamashta MA. Management of thrombosis and pregnancy loss in the antiphospholipid syndrome. Lupus 1998;2(Suppl 7):S162–5.
[7] Amengual O, Atsumi T, Khamashta MA, et al. Advances in antiphospholipid (Hughes') syndrome. Ann Acad Med Singap 1998;27:61–6.
[8] Bick RL. Antiphospholipid thrombosis syndromes: etiology, pathophysiology, diagnosis and management. Int J Hematol 1997;65:193–8.
[9] Bick RL, Baker WF. The antiphospholipid and thrombosis syndromes. Med Clin North Am 1994;78:667–84.
[10] Bick RL, Arun B, Frenkel EP. Antiphospholipid thrombosis syndromes. Haemostasis 1999;29:111–34.
[11] Festin MR, Limson GM, Maruo T. Autoimmune causes of recurrent pregnancy loss. Kobe J Med Sci 1997;43:143–57.
[12] Roussev RG, Kaider BD, Price DE, et al. Laboratory evaluation of women experiencing reproductive failure. Am J of Reproductive Immunology (Copenhagen) 1996;35:415–20.
[13] Oshiro BT, Silver RM, Scott JR, et al. Antiphospholipid antibodies and fetal death. Obstet Gynecol 1996;87:489–93.
[14] Granger KA, Farquharson RG. Obstetric outcome in antiphospholipid syndrome. Lupus 1997;6:509–13.
[15] Borrelli AL, Brillante M, Borzacchiello C, et al. Hemocoagulative pathology and immunological recurrent abortion. Clin Exp Obstet Gynecol 1997;24:39–40.
[16] Hellan M, Kuhnel E, Speiser W, et al. Familial lupus anticoagulant: a case report and review of the literature. Blood Coagul Fibrinolysis 1998;9:195–200.
[17] Ogasawara M, Aoki K, Matsuura E, et al. Anti beta-2-glycoprotein I antibodies and lupus anticoagulant in patients with recurrent pregnancy loss: prevalence and clinical significance. Lupus 1996;5:587–92.
[18] Zangari M, Lockwood CJ, Scher J, et al. Prothrombin activation fragment (F1.2) is increased in pregnant patients with antiphospholipid antibodies. Thromb Res 1997;85:177–83.
[19] Aznar J, Factor V. Leiden and antibodies against phospholipids and protein S in a young woman with recurrent thromboses and abortion. Haematologica 1999;84:80–4.
[20] Aznar J, Villa P, Espana F, et al. Activated protein C resistance phenotype in patients with antiphospholipid antibodies. J Lab Clin Med 1997;130:202–8.
[21] Schultz DR. Antiphospholipid antibodies: basic immunology and assays. Semin Arthritis Rheum 1997;26:724–39.
[22] Amengual O, Atsumi T, Khamashta MA, et al. The role of the tissue factor pathway in the hypercoagulable state in patients with the antiphospholipid syndrome. Thromb Haemost 1998;79:276–81.

[23] Martini A, Ravelli A. The clinical significance of antiphospholipid antibodies. Ann Med 1997;29:159–63.
[24] Bussen SS, Steck T. Thyroid antibodies and their relation to antithrombin antibodies, anticardiolipin antibodies and lupus anticoagulant in women with recurrent spontaneous abortions (antithyroid, anticardiolipin and antithrombin autoantibodies and lupus anticoagulant in habitual aborters). Eur J Obstet Gynecol Reprod Biol 1997;74:139–43.
[25] Rand JH, Wu XX. Antibody-mediated disruption of the annexin-V antithrombotic shield: a new mechanism for thrombosis in the antiphospholipid syndrome. Thromb Haemost 1999;82:649–54.
[26] Rand JH, Wu XX, Andree HA, et al. Antiphospholipid antibodies accelerate plasma coagulation by inhibiting annexin-V binding to phospholipids: a "lupus procoagulant" phenomenon. Blood 1998;92:1652–60.
[27] Rauch J. Lupus anticoagulant antibodies: recognition of phospholipid-binding protein complexes. Lupus 1998;7(Suppl 2):S29–33.
[28] Rote NS, Vogt E, DeVere G, et al. The role of placental trophoblast in the pathophysiology of the antiphospholipid antibody syndrome. Am J of Reproductive Immunology (Copenhagen) 1998;39:125–36.
[29] Vogt E, Ng AK, Rote NS. Antiphosphatidylserine antibody removes annexin-V and facilitates the binding of prothrombin at the surface of a choriocarcinoma model of trophoblast differentiation. Am J Obstet Gynecol 1997;177:964–72.
[30] Lakasing L, Campa JS, Poston R, et al. Normal expression of tissue factor, thrombomodulin, and annexin V in placentas from women with antiphospholipid syndrome. Am J Obstet Gynecol 1999;181:180–9.
[31] Siaka C, Lambert M, Caron C, et al. Low prevalence of anti-annexin V antibodies in antiphospholipid syndrome with fetal loss. Revue de Medecine Interne 1999;20:762–5.
[32] Kaburaki J, Kuwana M, Yamamoto M, et al. Clinical significance of anti-annexin V antibodies in patients with systemic lupus erythematosus. Am J Hematol 1997;54:209–13.
[33] Eschwege V, Peynaud-Debayle E, Wolf M, et al. Prevalence of antiphospholipid-related antibodies in unselected patients with history of venous thrombosis. Blood Coagul Fibrinolysis 1998;9:429–34.
[34] Silver RM, Pierangeli SS, Edwin SS, et al. Pathogenic antibodies in women with obstetric features of antiphospholipid syndrome who have negative test results for lupus anticoagulant and anticardiolipin antibodies. Am J Obstet Gynecol 1997;176:628–33.
[35] Branch DW, Silver R, Pierangeli S, et al. Antiphospholipid antibodies other than lupus anticoagulant and anticardiolipin antibodies in women with recurrent pregnancy loss, fertile controls, and antiphospholipid syndrome. Obstet Gynecol 1997;89:549–55.
[36] Bick RL, Hoppensteadt D. Recurrent miscarriage syndrome and infertility due to blood coagulation/platelet defects: a review and update. Clin Appl Thromb Hemost 2005;11: 1–13.
[37] Toschi V, Motta A, Costelli C, et al. High prevalence of antiphosphatidylinositol antibodies in young patients with cerebral ischemia of undetermined cause. Stroke 1998;29: 1759–64.
[38] FDA MedWatch. Lovenox (enoxaparin sodium) injection [January 9, 2002: Aventis]: warnings FDA MedWatch 1/9/2002. Available at: http://www.fda.gov/medwatch/SAFETY/2002/jan02.htm#lovenox. Accessed January 2, 2002.
[39] Brown HL. Antiphospholipid antibodies and recurrent pregnancy loss. Clin Obstet Gynecol 1991;34:17–26.
[40] Perino A, Barba G, Cimino C, et al. Immunological problems in the recurrent abortion syndrome. Acta Eur Fertil 1989;20:199–202.
[41] Many A, Pauzner R, Carp H, et al. Treatment of patients with antiphospholipid antibodies during pregnancy. Am J Reprod Immunol 1992;28:216–8.
[42] Lubbe WF, Liggins GC. Role of lupus anticoagulant and autoimmunity in recurrent fetal loss. Semin Reprod Endocrinol 1988;6:181–90.

[43] Lin Q. Investigation of the association between autoantibodies and recurrent abortions. Chinese J Obstet Gynecol 1993;28:674–9.
[44] Cowchock FS, Reece EA, Balaban D, et al. Repeated fetal losses associated with antiphospholipid antibodies: a collaborative randomized trial comparing prednisone with low-dose heparin treatment. Am J Obstet Gynecol 1992;166:1318–23.
[45] Landy HJ, Kessler C, Kelly WK, et al. Obstetric performance in patients with the lupus anticoagulant and/or anticardiolipin antibodies. Am J Perinatol 1992;9:146–51.
[46] Semprini AE, Vucetich A, Garbo S, et al. Effect of prednisone and heparin treatment in 14 patients with poor reproductive efficiency related to lupus anticoagulant. Fetal Ther 1989;4(Suppl 1):73–6.
[47] Rosove MH, Tabsh K, Wasserstrum N, et al. Heparin therapy for pregnant women with lupus anticoagulant or anticardiolipin antibodies. Obstet Gynecol 1990;75:630–4.
[48] Kutteh WH, Ermel LD. A clinical trial for the treatment of the antiphospholipid antibody associated recurrent pregnancy loss with lower dose heparin and aspirin. Am J Reprod Immunol 1996;35:402–7.
[49] Parke A. The role of IVIG in the management of patients with antiphospholipid antibodies and recurrent pregnancy losses. In: Ballow M, editor. IVIG Therapy Today. Totowa (NJ): Humana Press, Inc.; 1992. p. 105–18.

Antiphospholipid Antibodies and Malignancy

Chi Pham, MD, Yu-Min Shen, MD*

The University of Texas Southwestern Medical Center at Dallas, 5323 Harry Hines Boulevard, Dallas, TX 75390-8852, USA

Antiphospholipid antibody syndrome is characterized clinically by venous or arterial thrombosis, recurrent fetal loss, or placental insufficiency in women. The diagnosis requires the persistent laboratory evidence of antibodies to phospholipids or plasma proteins that have affinity to the negatively charged phospholipids [1]. These include lupus anticoagulant detected by prolongation of phospholipid-dependent clotting assays, and antibodies detected by solid-phase immunoassays (ELISA) such as anticardiolipin antibodies and anti-β_2-glycoprotein I antibodies [2]. These first were described in patients who had systemic lupus erythematosus (SLE) [3], but they now are known to be associated with other systemic autoimmune diseases, including rheumatoid arthritis, systemic sclerosis, Sjögren's syndrome, and systemic vasculitis [4]. In addition to thrombosis and pregnancy complications, antiphospholipid antibodies also are seen in patients who have chronic infections, especially those secondary to hepatitis C virus [5,6] and HIV [7]. Antiphospholipid antibodies also can occur because of treatment with certain medications such as interferon [5,8]. Recently, antiphospholipid antibodies have been reported in conjunction with various solid and hematologic malignancies [9,10].

Numerous healthy individuals also harbor the antiphospholipid antibodies without any evidence of an underlying disease process. In a study of 552 asymptomatic healthy volunteers, it was noted that up to 9.4% tested positive for anticardiolipin antibody with 1.4% showing persistence of these antibodies on repeat testing [11].

CANCER AND HYPERCOAGULABILITY

Since the first description by Armand Trousseau of the association between thrombophlebitis and malignancy, it has been accepted that patients who have cancer are at a much higher risk of developing thromboembolic disease than the normal population [12]. In a large population-based, case-controlled

*Corresponding author. E-mail address: yu-min.shen@utsouthwestern.edu (Y-M Shen).

study, the Dutch demonstrated that the risk of venous thrombosis was increased sevenfold in patients who had malignancy compared with normal controls. The risk of thrombosis was highest in patients who had hematological malignancies, followed by lung cancer and gastrointestinal cancer [13]. A Medicare claim-based study of over 8 million patients also showed that the percentage of patients who had deep venous thrombosis and pulmonary embolism was slightly higher for patients who had malignancy compared with those without malignancy [14]. Although thromboembolic events often are seen at the time of cancer diagnosis or shortly thereafter, they also can precede the cancer diagnosis by months to years [15,16]. A Swedish study of 3795 patients suspected to have venous thrombosis showed that among 1383 patients with venography-confirmed thrombosis, 66 developed cancer in the first 6 months of follow-up compared with 37 patients without venographic evidence of thrombosis [17].

The mechanism underlying the prothrombotic state of malignancy is a complex interplay between the tumor cells and host cells, such that the delicate balance between coagulation and fibrinolysis is disrupted [18]. Recent advances have established that the essential factors of hemostasis participate directly in cancer growth and progression, in addition to their known hemostatic properties. These include tissue factor, cancer procoagulant, thrombin, tissue type, and urokinase plasminogen activators, plasminogen activator inhibitor 1 and 2. The effects of these coagulation factors contribute to the tumor cells' ability to proliferate, migrate, and induce proteolysis and permeability [19]. Observations that therapy with unfractionated heparin and low molecular weight heparins in cancer patients may offer survival benefit as anticancer drugs have generated renewed interest in this field and lend support to the laboratory data [20–22].

Recently, a series of case reports have suggested that antiphospholipid antibodies also may play a role in the thrombotic predisposition of malignancy. There are several possible theories as to the generation of antiphospholipid antibodies in the setting of malignancy [23]:

> Production of autoantibodies by immune system in response to tumor antigens
> Production of monoclonal antibodies with lupus anticoagulant and anticardiolipin activities
> Secretion of anticardiolipin antibody from tumor cells

The exact mechanism(s) by which antiphospholipid antibody leads to thrombosis remain an active area of investigation. Because many steps of the coagulation cascade take place on negatively charged phospholipid surfaces, antiphospholipid antibodies potentially could act at any level to disrupt normal hemostasis. One may speculate that antibodies to prothrombin may have an anticoagulant effect, whereas antibodies to protein C and annexin V may impair normal control of coagulation [24,25]. Recent advances in the understanding of the pathophysiology of antiphospholipid syndrome have centered on the dimerization of β_2-glycoprotein I on the phospholipid membrane as a result of antiphospholipid antibody binding, which then leads to receptor-mediated platelet activation and up-regulation of procoagulant properties on endothelial cells [26].

PREVALENCE

Although antiphospholipid antibodies usually are seen in association with thrombosis, they also can be detected in asymptomatic healthy volunteers as discussed previously [11]. The incidence of antiphospholipid antibodies is noted to be in the range of 4.5% to 9.4% in the healthy young population based on various studies [11,27]. The incidence, however, increases dramatically with age. A study of 64 healthy elderly patients with mean age of 81 years showed that 51.6% tested positive for anticardiolipin antibodies of the IgG and IgM isotopes [28]. The limitation of most of these studies is that the volunteers were tested only once. The definition of antiphospholipid syndrome requires the persistence of the antibodies measured at least 12 weeks apart [1]. It is not known what the true incidence of such antibodies is when restricted to only subjects with their persistence on repeat testing.

The incidence of antiphospholipid antibodies and the diagnosis of antiphospholipid syndrome may be much higher in patients who have cancer. To evaluate this, a large French study tested the sera of 1014 consecutive patients admitted to the department of internal medicine for the presence of antiphospholipid antibodies. Seventy-two patients (7.1%) were noted to be positive for the antibodies at least once. Twenty-two patients (2.8%) fulfilled the criteria for antiphospholipid syndrome. Fourteen (63.6%) of these 22 patients were diagnosed with a malignancy [29]. Similarly, several case series of patients with known cancer also demonstrated the high incidence of antiphospholipid antibodies. A case–control study of 145 patients who had cancer showed that higher levels of IgG anti-cardiolipin antibody were found in patients with malignancy when compared with the controlled population ($P<.02$). Twenty patients with anticardiolipin antibodies had evidence of thromboembolic disease; most of them had solid malignancy, including lung, breast, prostate, stomach, colon, gynecological, bladder, and others [30]. Higher incidence of antiphospholipid antibodies also has been described in patients who have hematological malignancies [31]. An Italian study of 100 consecutive patients who had lymphoma indicated that 27 patients tested positive for either anticardiolipin antibody or lupus anticoagulant [32]. This was much higher than the 8% prevalence seen in their age- and sex-matched control group. If restricted to patients who have malignancy and thrombosis, antiphospholipid antibodies may be seen in up to 60% of patients according to one study of Asian cancer patients [33]. Given the association between malignancy and antiphospholipid antibodies, antiphospholipid antibodies have been described in all types of neoplasm. Table 1 is compilation of the tumor types seen in two large series of patients who have antiphospholipid antibodies, and Table 2 shows the frequency of antiphospholipid antibodies in four series of cancer patients. Despite the high incidence of antiphospholipid antibodies in patients who have malignancies, it must be kept in mind that the average age of these patients is around

Table 1
Tumor types reported in two series of patients with antiphospholipid antibodies [9,36]

Hematologic malignancies	Number	Solid tumors	Number
B lymphoma	10	Central nervous system tumors	5
Lymphocytic lymphoma	4	Otorhinolaryngology tumors	8
Lymphoplasmacytoid lymphoma	1	Papillary thyroid carcinoma	1
Angiocentric lymphoma	1	Thyroid	3
Spleen lymphoma	8	Thymoma	1
Hairy cell leukemia	4	Tracheal carcinoma	1
Peripheral T lymphoma	1	Lung adenocarcinoma	6
Cutaneous T lymphoma	3	Nonsmall cell lung cancer	3
Non-Hodgkin lymphoma	15	Mesothelioma	1
Hodgkin's	3	Breast carcinoma	15
Multiple myeloma	3	Gastric carcinoma	1
Waldenstrom's macroglobulinemia	3	Cholangiocarcinoma	2
Monoclonal gammopathy	2	Hepatocarcinoma	2
Chronic lymphocytic leukemia	2	Colon carcinoma	6
Chronic myeloid leukemia	7	Carcinoid tumor	1
Acute leukemias	2	Uterine carcinoma	2
Acute lymphocytic leukemia	1	Cervix	2
Acute myeloid leukemia	3	Ovarian carcinoma	2
Myeloproliferative disorders	6	Renal cell	9
Lymphosarcoma	2	Prostatic adenocarcinoma	8
		Testicle	1
		Urinary tract	4
		Leiomyoblastoma	1
		Leiomyosarcoma	1
		Melanoma	6
		Skin	2
		Skin squamous cell carcinoma	1
		Unknown origin	6

60 years old [34]. As previously discussed, elderly individuals tend to have much higher rates of harboring these antibodies than the healthy normal population.

MANIFESTATION

Patients who have malignancy commonly are diagnosed as having antiphospholipid syndrome when they present with thrombotic events. These include both arterial and venous thrombosis. The most common venous events are deep venous thrombosis and pulmonary embolism, whereas the most common arterial events are myocardial infarction and cerebrovascular accident [35]. In a study by Miesbach and colleagues [36] of 58 patients who had neoplasia and antiphospholipid syndrome, arterial thrombosis was identified much more commonly than venous thrombosis. They also noted that patients who had solid malignancy were much more likely to have a thrombotic event compared with patients with a hematological or lymphoproliferative disorder ($P>.05$).

Table 2
Frequency of antiphospholipid antibodies in series of cancer patients

	LA	aCL IgG	aCL IgM	aCL IgG/M	aCL IgA	aβ2GPI IgG	aβ2GPI IgM	aβ2GPI IgA	aβ2GPI
All cancers									
Number positive	2	2	5		0	2	0	15	
Number tested	21	30	30		30	32	32	32	
Percent positive	9.5%	6.7%	16.7%		0%	6.25%	0%	46.875	
References	[33]	[33]	[33]		[33]	[33]	[33]	[33]	
Lymphoma (Hodgkin's and non-Hodgkin's)									
Number positive	19	4	11	25	5	1	14	19	12
Number tested	167	175	172	100	62	72	72	72	90
Percent positive	11.4%	2.3%	6.4%	25.0%	8.1%	1.4%	19.4%	26.4%	13.3%
References	[31,32]	[31,34]	[31,34]	[32]	[31]	[31]	[31]	[31]	[34]
Acute myeloid leukemia									
Number positive		11	6	8					
Number tested		37	37	37					
Percent positive		29.7%	16.2%	21.6%					
References		[53]	[53]	[53]					

Please note that the case series employed different inclusion criteria and laboratory methods.
Abbreviations: aCL, anti-cardiolipin antibody; aβ2GPI, anti-beta-2 glycoprotein I antibody; IgG/IgM, no distinction made between the two isotypes; LA, lupus anticoagulant.
Data from Refs. [31–34,53].

Others, however, have reported similar thrombotic complication rates in patients who have hematological malignancies. Pusterla and colleagues [32] demonstrated in a case-controlled study that in patients who had lymphoma, the rate of thrombosis was significantly higher in patients who had antiphospholipid antibodies than those without the antibodies (5.1% per year versus 0.75% per year, respectively).

There are case reports of other rare thrombotic manifestations in patients who have cancer and antiphospholipid antibodies. These include necrotizing leg ulcers [37], recurrent stent thrombosis [38], transverse myelitis [39], and nonbacterial thrombotic endocarditis [40]. The most feared complication is the catastrophic antiphospholipid antibody syndrome, or Asherson's syndrome. This syndrome is characterized by multiple sites of thromboses with multiorgan failure that is often fatal [41]. Several case reports of malignancy have been linked to catastrophic antiphospholipid syndrome [42,43], although it remains an extremely rare occurrence. According to one study, which consisted of 1000 patients with antiphospholipid syndrome, only 0.8% of patients had criteria for Asherson's syndrome [44].

It remains to be determined whether having antiphospholipid antibodies in the setting of malignancy indeed leads to a higher risk of thrombosis. In contrast to the previous studies, a study by Genvresse and colleagues [34] showed that 26.6% of patients with non-Hodgkin's lymphoma had evidence of elevated antiphospholipid antibodies, but none developed any thromboembolic event during 14 months of follow-up. Similarly, a study of four patients who had elevated IgG and IgM anticardiolipin antibody and lupus anticoagulant did not demonstrate any thromboembolic manifestation during the entire follow-up period [45]. At this point, the role antiphospholipid antibodies play in patients with malignancy is still controversial. It is unclear if these antibodies represent an epiphenomenon or contribute to the pathogenesis of thrombosis in patients who have malignancy.

ANTIPHOSPHOLIPID ANTIBODY AND PROGNOSIS

The Italian Registry of Antiphospholipid Antibodies followed 360 patients prospectively over 5 years to assess the natural history of antiphospholipid syndrome. With a median follow up of 3.9 years, the Italians noted four new cases of non-Hodgkin's lymphoma and one new case of breast cancer. For non-Hodgkin's lymphoma, the estimated event rate was 0.28% patient-year, which is much higher than the expected incidence of non-Hodgkin's lymphoma of 5 to 15 cases per 100,000 population per year. The study investigators concluded that antiphospholipid antibodies should be considered a risk factor for non-Hodgkin's lymphoma [46].

Treatment of the underlying malignancy often leads to the disappearance of antiphospholipid antibody [9,29]. In a report by Sciarra and colleagues [47], patients with acute myelogenous leukemia or non-Hodgkin's lymphoma who had elevated titers of antiphospholipid antibodies at diagnosis were shown to have undetectable antibody levels after treatment of their leukemia or lymphoma if they responded to the prescribed therapy. In contrast, the antibodies were persistent in those patients who did not respond. Furthermore, patients who responded and had disappearance of their antiphospholipid antibodies later were noted to have recurrence of the antibodies when their disease relapsed [47]. Some patients who tested negative for antiphospholipid antibodies were noted to be positive when their cancer progressed or became refractory to the treatment [48]. Thus, the presence of antiphospholipid antibodies may serve as a surrogate marker for disease status and response to therapy for hematologic malignancies.

Similar findings also were seen in patients who had solid tumors. In a report by Miesbach and colleagues [36], two patients who had colon carcinoma and antiphospholipid antibody were noted to have disappearance of the antiphospholipid antibody after effective treatment of their colon cancer. As long as the patients were in remission, the antiphospholipid testing remained negative. Despite the fact that they presented with clots initially, once the antiphospholipid antibody became undetectable, they did not have recurrence of the thrombotic event.

Even though the presence of antiphospholipid antibody is indicative of the persistence of the underlying malignancy, antiphospholipid antibody has not been correlated with tumor stage, age, performance status, or International Prognostic Index (IPI) score in the case of non-Hodgkin's lymphoma [31,34]. Antiphospholipid antibody, however, may serve as an independent prognostic variable in aggressive lymphoma. A study of patients who had non-Hodgkin's lymphoma showed that the 2-year survival was 90% plus or minus 5% for patients without antiphospholipid antibody at diagnosis compared with 63% plus or minus 11% for patients with an elevated antibody level ($P = .0025$) [31]. This observation requires validation with further studies.

SUMMARY

Presence of antiphospholipid antibodies is a significant thrombophilic risk factor with a high prevalence in patients who have malignancies [32]. Patients who harbor these antibodies may be at increased risk for thromboembolic complications [49]. The mechanism by which antiphospholipid antibody develops in the setting of malignancy is poorly understood. It is postulated that the antibodies may be a direct consequence of the tumor itself [50], a normal immune reaction to the tumor, or it also could be caused by specific cancer therapies [51]. The presence of antiphospholipid antibody does not predict the likelihood of response to treatment necessarily, nor does it affect prognosis, with the possible exception of high grade lymphomas. It may help in monitoring disease activity, because cancers in remission often are accompanied by disappearance of antiphospholipid antibody [47]. Manipulating the antibody levels with immunosuppressive therapy has not been shown to affect the thrombosis risk or its recurrence [52]. Patients should be treated only if they develop a thromboembolic event. Prospective studies should be conducted to elucidate these issues.

References

[1] Miyakis S, Lockshin MD, Atsumi T, et al. International consensus statement on an update of the classification criteria for definite antiphospholipid syndrome (APS). J Thromb Haemost 2006;4(2):295–306.
[2] Passam F, Krilis S. Laboratory tests for the antiphospholipid syndrome: current concepts. Pathology 2004;36:129–38.
[3] Conley CL. A hemorrhagic disorder caused by circulating anticoagulant in patients with disseminated lupus erythematosus. J Clin Invest 1952;31:621–2.
[4] Cervera R, Asherson RA. Clinical and epidemiological aspects in the antiphospholipid syndrome. Immunobiology 2003;207(1):5–11.
[5] Matsuda J, Saitoh N, Gotoh M, et al. High prevalence of antiphospholipid antibodies and antithyroglobulin antibody in patients with hepatitis C virus infection treated with interferon-alpha. Am J Gastroenterol 1995;90(7):1138–41.
[6] Prieto J, Yuste JR, Beloqui O, et al. Anticardiolipin antibodies in chronic hepatitis C: implication of hepatitis C virus as the cause of the antiphospholipid syndrome. Hepatology 1996;23(2):199–204.
[7] Uthman IW, Gharavi AE. Viral infections and antiphospholipid antibodies. Semin Arthritis Rheum 2002;31(4):256–63.
[8] Naldi L, Locati F, Finazzi G, et al. Antiphospholipid syndrome associated with immunotherapy for patients with melanoma. Cancer 1995;75(11):2784–5.
[9] Gomez-Puerta JA, Cervera R, Espinosa G, et al. Antiphospholipid antibodies associated with malignancies: clinical and pathological characteristics of 120 patients. Semin Arthritis Rheum 2006;35(5):322–32.
[10] Pugliese LBI, Pacifico E, Viola-Magni M, et al. Antiphospholipid antibodies in patients with cancer. Int J Immunopathol Pharmacol 2006;19(4):879–88.
[11] Vila P, Hernandez MC, Lopez-Fernandez MF, et al. Prevalence, follow-up, and clinical significance of the anticardiolipin antibodies in normal subjects. Thromb Haemost 1994;72(2):209–13.
[12] Sack GH Jr, Levin J, Bell WR. Trousseau's syndrome and other manifestations of chronic disseminated coagulopathy in patients with neoplasms: clinical, pathophysiologic, and therapeutic features. Medicine (Baltimore) 1977;56(1):1–37.
[13] Blom JW, Doggen CJ, Osanto S, et al. Malignancies, prothrombotic mutations, and the risk of venous thrombosis. JAMA 2005;293(6):715–22.
[14] Levitan N, Dowlati A, Remick SC, et al. Rates of initial and recurrent thromboembolic disease among patients with malignancy versus those without malignancy. Risk analysis using Medicare claims data. Medicine (Baltimore) 1999;78(5):285–91.
[15] White RH, Chew HK, Zhou H, et al. Incidence of venous thromboembolism in the year before the diagnosis of cancer in 528,693 adults. Arch Intern Med 2005;165(15):1782–7.
[16] Prandoni P, Lensing AW, Buller HR, et al. Deep vein thrombosis and the incidence of subsequent symptomatic cancer. N Engl J Med 1992;327(16):1128–33.
[17] Nordstrom M, Lindblad B, Anderson H, et al. Deep venous thrombosis and occult malignancy: an epidemiological study. BMJ 1994;308(6933):891–4.
[18] Gouin-Thibault I, Achkar A, Samama MM. The thrombophilic state in cancer patients. Acta Haematol 2001;106(1–2):33–42.
[19] Buller HR, van Doormaal FF, van Sluis GL, et al. Cancer and thrombosis: from molecular mechanisms to clinical presentations. J Thromb Haemost 2007;5(Suppl 1):246–54.
[20] Kakkar AK, Levine MN, Kadziola Z, et al. Low molecular weight heparin, therapy with dalteparin, and survival in advanced cancer: the fragmin advanced malignancy outcome study (FAMOUS). J Clin Oncol 2004;22(10):1944–8.
[21] Klerk CP, Smorenburg SM, Otten HM, et al. The effect of low molecular weight heparin on survival in patients with advanced malignancy. J Clin Oncol 2005;23(10):2130–5.

[22] Lee AY, Rickles FR, Julian JA, et al. Randomized comparison of low molecular weight heparin and coumarin derivatives on the survival of patients with cancer and venous thromboembolism. J Clin Oncol 2005;23(10):2123–9.
[23] Zuckerman E, Toubi E, Golan TD, et al. Increased thromboembolic incidence in anticardiolipin-positive patients with malignancy. Br J Cancer 1995;72(2):447–51.
[24] Hanly JG, Smith SA, Anderson D. Inhibition of annexin V binding to cardiolipin and thrombin generation in an unselected population with venous thrombosis. J Rheumatol 2003;30(9):1990–3.
[25] Rand JH, Wu XX, Quinn AS, et al. Human monoclonal antiphospholipid antibodies disrupt the annexin A5 anticoagulant crystal shield on phospholipid bilayers: evidence from atomic force microscopy and functional assay. Am J Pathol 2003;163(3):1193–200.
[26] Giannakopoulos B, Passam F, Rahgozar S, et al. Current concepts on the pathogenesis of the antiphospholipid syndrome. Blood 2007;109(2):422–30.
[27] Shi W, Krilis SA, Chong BH, et al. Prevalence of lupus anticoagulant and anticardiolipin antibodies in a healthy population. Aust N Z J Med 1990;20(3):231–6.
[28] Manoussakis MN, Tzioufas AG, Silis MP, et al. High prevalence of anticardiolipin and other autoantibodies in a healthy elderly population. Clin Exp Immunol 1987;69(3):557–65.
[29] Schved JF, Dupuy-Fons C, Biron C, et al. A prospective epidemiological study on the occurrence of antiphospholipid antibody: the Montpellier Antiphospholipid (MAP) Study. Haemostasis 1994;24(3):175–82.
[30] Armas JB, Dantas J, Mendonca D, et al. Anticardiolipin and antinuclear antibodies in cancer patients—a case control study. Clin Exp Rheumatol 2000;18(2):227–32.
[31] Bairey O, Blickstein D, Monselise Y, et al. Antiphospholipid antibodies may be a new prognostic parameter in aggressive non-Hodgkin's lymphoma. Eur J Haematol 2006;76(5):384–91.
[32] Pusterla S, Previtali S, Marziali S, et al. Antiphospholipid antibodies in lymphoma: prevalence and clinical significance. Hematol J 2004;5(4):341–6.
[33] Yoon KH, Wong A, Shakespeare T, et al. High prevalence of antiphospholipid antibodies in Asian cancer patients with thrombosis. Lupus 2003;12(2):112–6.
[34] Genvresse I, Luftner D, Spath-Schwalbe E, et al. Prevalence and clinical significance of anticardiolipin and anti-beta2-glycoprotein-I antibodies in patients with non-Hodgkin's lymphoma. Eur J Haematol 2002;68(2):84–90.
[35] Shortell CK, Ouriel K, Green RM, et al. Vascular disease in the antiphospholipid syndrome: a comparison with the patient population with atherosclerosis. J Vasc Surg 1992;15(1):158–65 [discussion: 165–6].
[36] Miesbach W, Scharrer I, Asherson R. Thrombotic manifestations of the antiphospholipid syndrome in patients with malignancies. Clin Rheumatol 2006;25(6):840–4.
[37] Andrejevic S, Bonaci-Nikolic B, Bukilica M, et al. Purpura and leg ulcers in a patient with cryoglobulinaemia, non-Hodgkin's lymphoma, and antiphospholipid syndrome. Clin Exp Dermatol 2003;28(2):151–3.
[38] Muir DF, Stevens A, Napier-Hemy RO, et al. Recurrent stent thrombosis associated with lupus anticoagulant due to renal cell carcinoma. Int J Cardiovasc Intervent 2003;5(1):44–6.
[39] Carter D, Olchovsky D, Yonath H, et al. Simultaneous deep vein thrombosis and transverse myelitis with negative serology as a first sign of antiphospholipid syndrome: a case report and review of the literature. Clin Rheumatol 2006;25(5):756–8.
[40] Gonzalez Quintela A, Candela MJ, Vidal C, et al. Nonbacterial thrombotic endocarditis in cancer patients. Acta Cardiol 1991;46(1):1–9.
[41] Asherson RA, Cervera R, Piette JC, et al. Catastrophic antiphospholipid syndrome: clues to the pathogenesis from a series of 80 patients. Medicine (Baltimore) 2001;80(6):355–77.
[42] Soltesz P, Szekanecz Z, Vegh J, et al. Catastrophic antiphospholipid syndrome in cancer. Haematologia (Budap) 2000;30(4):303–11.

[43] Yamamoto T, Ito M, Nagata S, et al. Catastrophic exacerbation of antiphospholipid syndrome after lung adenocarcinoma biopsy. J Rheumatol 2000;27(8):2035–7.
[44] Cervera R, Piette JC, Font J, et al. Antiphospholipid syndrome: clinical and immunologic manifestations and patterns of disease expression in a cohort of 1000 patients. Arthritis Rheum 2002;46(4):1019–27.
[45] Miesbach W, Scharrer I, Asherson RA. High titres of IgM-antiphospholipid antibodies are unrelated to pathogenicity in patients with non-Hodgkin's lymphoma. Clin Rheumatol 2007;26(1):95–7.
[46] Finazzi G. The Italian registry of antiphospholipid antibodies. Haematologica 1997;82(1):101–5.
[47] Sciarra A, Stasi R, Stipa E, et al. [Antiphospholipid antibodies: their prevalence, clinical significance and correlation with cytokine levels in acute myeloid leukemia and non-Hodgkin's lymphoma]. Recenti Prog Med 1995;86(2):57–62.
[48] Stasi R, Stipa E, Masi M, et al. Antiphospholipid [in Italian] antibodies: prevalence, clinical significance, and correlation to cytokine levels in acute myeloid leukemia and non-Hodgkin's lymphoma. Thromb Haemost 1993;70(4):568–72.
[49] Palosuo T, Virtamo J, Haukka J, et al. High antibody levels to prothrombin imply a risk of deep venous thrombosis and pulmonary embolism in middle-aged men—a nested case–control study. Thromb Haemost 1997;78(4):1178–82.
[50] Sawamura M, Yamaguchi S, Murakami H, et al. Multiple autoantibody production in a patient with splenic lymphoma. Ann Hematol 1994;68(5):251–4.
[51] Becker JC, Winkler B, Klingert S, et al. Antiphospholipid syndrome associated with immunotherapy for patients with melanoma. Cancer 1994;73(6):1621–4.
[52] Joseph RE, Radhakrishnan J, Appel GB. Antiphospholipid antibody syndrome and renal disease. Curr Opin Nephrol Hypertens 2001;10(2):175–81.
[53] Lossos IS, Bogomolski-Yahalom V, Matzner Y. Anticardiolipin antibodies in acute myeloid leukemia: prevalence and clinical significance. Am J Hematol 1998;57(2):139–43.

Antiphospholipid Syndromes in Infectious Diseases

Navin M. Amin, MD, DTM&H[a,b,c,d,*]

[a]David Geffen School of Medicine, University of California, Los Angeles, 10833 Le Conte Avenue, Los Angeles, CA 90095, USA
[b]University of California Irvine Medical Center, Bld. 200, Suite 512, Route 81, Orange, CA 92868-3298, USA
[c]Stanford University, 300 Pasteur Drive, Stanford, CA 94305, USA
[d]Department of Family Medicine, Kern Medical Center, Bakersfield, CA, USA

Antiphospholipid syndrome (APS), or the classic "Hughes syndrome," first described between 1983 and 1996, is a systemic disorder, autoimmune in nature, characterized by various vaso-occlusive and hemocytopenic manifestations, predominately with multiple arterial or venous thrombosis, recurrent spontaneous abortions and fetal wastage, mild to moderate thrombocytopenia, hemolytic anemia, positive Coombs test, pulmonary hypertension, arthritis, central nervous system manifestations (stroke, transverse myelitis, Guillain-Barre syndrome), and detection of elevated levels of antiphospholipid antibodies (aPL), namely anticardiolipin antibodies (aCL) or lupus anticoagulant (LA) [1,2]. It can be a primary clinical disorder, commonly associated with connective tissue disease like systemic lupus erythematosus (41.2%) [3] and other autoimmune diseases like rheumatoid arthritis and Sjögren's syndrome.

Many other conditions can be associated with aPL but are not necessarily associated with thrombotic manifestations. aPL may occur in various infections, in certain malignancies like hairy cell leukemia, and with exposure to various drugs like chlorpromazine, quinine, quinidine, hydralazine, procainamide, phenytoin, and interferon-alpha. aPL in these circumstances are not necessarily pathogenic but should be considered in differential diagnosis of APS [4].

HISTORICAL BACKGROUND

aPL have been strongly related to various infections. These antibodies were detected for the first time in sera from a patient who had syphilis. In 1906, Wassermann used saline extract of the liver and spleen of a fetus with congenital

*1111 Columbus Street, Suite 1200, Bakersfield, CA 93305. E-mail address: aminn@kernmedctr.com

syphilis as an antigen in a complement fixation test and demonstrated a positive reaction with syphilitic sera. The antibody was called Wassermann reagin and was introduced as a serologic test for syphilis [4–6]. The antigenic component of this test was isolated and identified as a phospholipids-cardiolipin, marking the beginning of detection of aPL in various infections.

PATHOGENIC HYPOTHESIS

aPL have been detected and strongly associated with numerous microbial and viral infections, although a pathogenic role for these antibodies has not usually been obvious, except in a few cases.

aPL will bind to phospholipid by a cofactor known as B2 glycoprotein I (B_2 GPI), a glycoprotein with anticoagulant properties predominantly seen in autoimmune diseases, resulting in thrombotic manifestations of APS [6]. In other situations, like varied infection or drug-induced aPL production, a cofactor was not needed to enhance binding and therefore did not cause typical thrombotic symptoms [7,8].

The two types of aPL were referred to as "autoimmune" and "infectious." This distinction, however, has subsequently been found to be absolute. Recent postulation is that aPL associated with infection do not possess anti–B_2 GPI activity and are not associated with thrombotic complications. However, in leprosy patients, investigators have found increased levels of anti–B_2 GPI antibodies that were associated with thrombosis [9]. Similarly, aCL binding characteristics were seen in human parvovirus B_{19} infection, which led to the hypothesis that infections may be a trigger for the induction of pathogenic aPL in certain predisposed subjects. The B_2 GPI induced by infections may bind to "self" aPL, thus forming an immunogenic complex against the aPL that are then produced. What constitutes the predisposition is not known, but clearly, genetic factors play a major role. The antibodies produced by infectious "triggers" are therefore heterogeneous in their dependency on B_2 GPI and few may resemble the autoimmune type [10]. Microbial agents or viruses can induce autoimmune diseases by various mechanisms [11]. For example, proteins of certain infectious agents can act as polyclonal activators on unique lymphocyte subsets. Viruses can preferentially infect and destroy a particular T-cell subset, leading to an imbalance in the immune response. In other instances, infectious agents can up-regulate Th1 cytokines, thereby increasing the selected expression of molecules such as MHC glycoproteins. Microbes can also direct the release of cytokines and chemokines, which can act as growth, differentiation, or chemotactic factors for different Th populations and regulate MHC class I and class II molecules [12]. The healthy immune system is tolerant of the molecules of which the body is composed. However, among major antigens recognized during various bacterial, viral, and parasitic diseases, many belong to conserved protein families sharing extensive sequence identity or conformation fits with the host's molecules, namely molecular mimicry [13]. Antigenic similarity between antigens of infectious agents and host tissues might trigger an immune response against the shared determinants. As a result, the tolerance to autoantigens breaks down and the pathogen-specific immune response that is generated cross-reacts with host structures to cause tissue damage and disease. Molecular mimicry between common pathogens and B_2 GPI may be one of the main causes of the induction of APS [13,14].

INFECTIONS AND ANTIPHOSPHOLIPID ANTIBODIES

aPL may be demonstrated during the course of many infections, in addition to occurring in conditions such as systemic lupus erythematosus, primary APS, and various other rheumatic diseases. Among the predominant aPL in patients who have various infections is a propensity for IgM isotype aCL. An increase in IgG isotype may also be detected. LA, either alone or with aCL, is encountered in few infections. Cryoglobulins, rheumatoid factor, and antinuclear antibodies are detected at some time during the course of acute illness [3,6,15].

Many infections may be associated with an increase in aPL (Box 1); however, in some, these increases may be accompanied by clinical manifestations of APS [6,16,17]. Skin infection (18%), HIV infection (17%), pneumonia (14%), hepatitis C virus (HCV) (13%), and urinary tract (10%) have constituted the most common infections found as triggering factors. In a few cases, more than one agent or organ was identified as the source.

ANTIPHOSPHOLIPID ANTIBODIES IN VARIOUS INFECTIONS
Antiphospholipid Antibodies in Hepatitis C Infection

Hepatitis C is a hepatotropic and lymphotropic virus that is associated with hepatic and extrahepatic manifestations [15,18]. HCV tends to induce nonspecific autoimmune reactions, as demonstrated by a high prevalence of various non–organ-specific autoantibodies usually in low titers, including antinuclear, smooth muscle, antineutrophil, and liver–kidney microsomal antibodies [18].

aCL have been widely reported [19–21] in HCV infection. The prevalence of these antibodies ranges from 3.3% to 46%, as reported in 15 studies with 1475 patients [15]. The high variation in aCL prevalence can be attributed to the laboratory methods used and to the design of the studies. For instance, it is important to know whether a commercial enzyme-linked immunosorbent assay (ELISA) kit or a homemade, standardized, internationally accepted ELISA was used to determine aCL.

In addition, no relationship between HCV and APS was established from these studies [15] and no clinical manifestation of APS was reported in aCL- and HCV-positive patients before or during follow-up visits [22–24]. aCL detected in the patients who had HCV infections were of the nonthrombogenic type, which means that they were cofactor independent [18,19,25]. This finding, along with the absence of LA activity, justifies the lack of clinical manifestations of APS in HCV-infected patients. Prieto and colleagues [20] found 22% of subjects with cirrhosis-related portal hypertension, thrombocytopenia, and previous thrombotic events to have higher titers of aCL [19,20]. Cirrhosis, whatever its cause, is frequently associated with the presence of nonpathogenic aCL [19,26].

Box 1: Antiphospholipid antibodies in various infections

Viral
Cytomegalovirus
HIV
Parvovirus B_{19}
Vaccina
Mumps
Human T-lymphotropic virus-1
Epstein-Barr virus
Hepatitis C
Varicella
Adenovirus
Rubella

Bacterial
Gram-positives
- Streptococcus pyogenes
- Staphylococcus aureus

Gram-negatives
- Salmonella Typhi
- Klebsiella pneumonie
- Shigella dysenteriae
- Helicobacter pylori

Atypicals
- Mycoplasma pneumoniae
- Mycoplasma penetrans

Mycobacterials
- Mycobacterium tuberculosis
- Mycobacterium leprae

Spirochetes
- Treponema palladium
- Borrelia burgdorferi
- Leptospira

Rickettsiae
- Coxiella burnetii

Parasites
- Leishmania
- Toxoplasma
- Malaria

Adapted from Asherson R A, Cervera R. Antiphospholipid antibodies and infections. Ann Rheum Dis 2003;62:388–93; with permission.

However, several cases of patients who had HCV and thrombosis have been reported. One patient who had thalassemia and HCV and who developed thrombosis [27] had aCL and LA present. Baid and colleagues [28], studying aCL and renal allograft thrombosis in 18 patients who had HCV positivity before transplant, found that renal microangiopathy with aCL positivity had developed in 5 patients, compared with only 1 of 13 without angiopathy. Malwick and colleagues [29] also reported a case of a 54-year-old man who had a chronic HCV infection and a high level of aCL, who developed a lacunar brain infarction [29,30].

In summary, the prevalence of aCL in patients who have HCV infection is found at a higher proportion than in controlled groups. In most cases, the titers of these antibodies are low, cofactor independent, and unrelated to APS manifestations. A positive correlation between HCV and APS seems unlikely; therefore, it is not recommended to test for HCV in patients who have APS. In a few patients, thrombotic complications may occur.

Antiphospholipid Antibodies in HIV Infection

HIV, a retrovirus, causes abnormalities of T- and B-cell function that result in development of various autoimmune phenomena of unknown but pathogenic significance. In 1986, Bloom and colleagues [31] first documented the presence of LA in 40% of AIDS patients and in 43% of asymptomatic HIV-positive individuals (in which they may be transient) [17,31]. In 1992, Argov and colleagues [32] reported the association of aCL with HIV infection in male homosexuals [16,32]. Since then, many studies have alluded to a high prevalence of aCL in patients who have HIV (range 12%–67%) [33–36]. In contrast, anti-B_2 GPI antibodies are rarely detected in HIV patients, which indicates that aCL in such individuals have characteristics of the natural type, not the pathogenic [37] variety. aCL in HIV patients have been associated with the presence of cerebral perfusion defects and transient neurologic deficit, but association with thrombosis is uncommon, even with high aCL titers [38].

Antibodies against phospholipids other than cardiolipin, such as phosphatidylserine, phosphatidylinositol, and phosphatidylcholine, have also been detected in HIV-infected patients [36]. According to Guerin and colleagues [39], who found LA positivity in 72% and aCL positivity of 67% in their HIV patients, the detection of antibodies to prothrombin and B_2 GPI is significantly less when compared with patients who have definite APS. Thus, in HIV infection, both types of aCL-nonpathogenic (non–B_2 GPI dependent) and pathogenic (B_2 GPI dependent) antibodies may be detected [6]. Petrovas and colleagues [35] demonstrated that aPL reactivity does not correlate with the disease duration or stage of HIV infection or with history of pneumocystis pneumonia or coinfection with HCV. aCL did not appear to be a prognostic marker in HIV-infected subjects [40]. A significant decrease of aCL binding after treatment with urea and sodium chloride was observed in the sera of HIV-infected patients when compared with APS patients, indicating that aCL from HIV patients have a low resistance to dissociating agents [41].

In patients who have HIV or AIDS, thrombosis occurs frequently, including peripheral vein, pulmonary embolism [42], retinal vein [43], cerebral vein [44], portal vein [45], mesenteric [46] occlusions, and testicular vessel [47]. Bosson and colleagues [48] reported a patient who had both arterial and venous thromboembolism. In 1994, Thirumalai and colleagues [49] reported the presence of aCL and stroke in an HIV-positive patient. In 1993, Cappell and colleagues [50] reported a case of 33-year-old woman with AIDS who had a cerebrovascular accident and developed splenic infarction. In 1993, Belmonte and colleagues [51] documented three cases of avascular necrosis of bone associated with elevated aPL. Opportunistic infections, particularly with coexisting cytomegalovirus (CMV), or, on occasion, pneumocystis, have been associated with thrombosis [52].

In summary, therefore, it seems that the pathogenesis of thrombotic complications in HIV-infected patients and patients who have AIDS is multifactorial, with aPL playing a role in selected patients only. Although thrombotic complications encountered with aPL positivity have been reported from various centers, their frequency remains low at present. Lipid disturbances associated with antiretroviral therapy may be an additional cause of these complications.

Antiphospholipid Antibodies in Cytomegalovirus Infection

IgG and IgM isotypes of aCL have been detected in CMV infections. Labarca and colleagues [53] described a healthy young man who developed mesenteric and femoropopliteal thrombosis during the course of CMV infection. He responded well to treatment with anticoagulants; 6 months after the onset of APS, IgM and IgG aCL titers declined. A similar case with transitory manifestation of APS was reported by Uthman and colleagues [54] in 1999. Dual viral infection with CMV and HIV have frequently resulted in thrombotic manifestations of APS [44], including digital infarcts [55].

Within the last year, a high prevalence (56%) of aPL was reported in CMV infection among patients who received unrelated bone marrow and cord blood allogenic stem cell transplantation for hematologic malignancies [56]. No association was noted between these antibodies and the clinical expression of autoimmunity.

Antiphospholipid Antibodies in Parvovirus B_{19} Infection

Infection with parvovirus B_{19} was associated with predominantly IgG antibodies against the negatively charged phospholipids, cardiolipin and phosphatidylserine, which were B_2 GPI dependent, as seen in patients who have systemic lupus erythematosus [10]. Unlike antibodies from patients who have other viral infections (like HCV and HIV) or from those with syphilis, parvovirus infection was associated with aCL and increased their binding to antigen in the presence of B_2 GPI as a binding cofactor, resulting in thrombotic manifestations.

Antiphospholipid Antibodies in Varicella Virus Infection

Transient elevation of IgM and IgG aCL and LA is detected in patients who have acute varicella infection. In a few cases, raised anti–B_2 GPI antibodies were observed with thrombotic manifestations. Uthman and colleagues [57] reported a 16-year-old young man with iliofemoral thrombosis 1 week after chicken pox infection. Manco-Johnson and colleagues [58], studying seven children with varicella, documented an association with thrombosis in four who had elevated aPL.

Antiphospholipid Antibodies in Human T-Lymphotropic Virus-1 Infection

Human T-lymphotropic virus-1 (HTLV-1) is a retrovirus commonly detected as an asymptomatic infection in blood donors. With prolonged infection with HTLV-1, some patients can develop tropical spastic paraparesis. In such individuals, IgA aCL titers are frequently elevated, as reported by Faghiri and colleagues [59].

Antiphospholipid Antibodies in Epstein-Barr Virus Infection

Sorice and colleagues [60], in their study, found that 30% of the patients who had infectious mononucleosis due to Epstein-Barr virus infection were positive for aCL. These antibodies (meaning aCL) were often present with anti-cofactor protein antibodies (B_2GPI), but the prevalence of this combination is low. aCL and anti-cofactor protein antibodies disappeared after 12 to 15 months of Epstein-Barr virus infections.

Yamazaki and colleagues [61] reported a single case of a 25-year-old woman who had Epstein-Barr virus infection and developed deep vein thrombosis and pulmonary embolus with elevated LA and aCL titers. After 6 months, antibody titers reverted to normal.

Antiphospholipid Antibodies in Bacterial Infections

Many bacterial infections demonstrate the presence of aPL; however, these increases in aPL are usually not associated with thrombotic events, and B_2 GPI dependence is usually negative. The most common isotypes of aCL seen in various bacterial infections are IgG and IgM, with some cases having IgA (Table 1).

Table 1
Prevalence and isotypes of anticardiolipin antibodies in various infections

Infection	Frequency (%)	Isotype
Leprosy	33–67	IgG, IgM, IgA
Tuberculosis	27–53	IgG, IgM
Mycoplasma	20–53	IgG, IgM, IgA
Streptococcus	80	IgG, IgM, IgA
Salmonella	60	IgG, IgM, IgA
Staphylococcus	43	IgG, IgM, IgA
Leptospira	50	IgG
Borrelia	14–41	IgG, IgM
Coxiella burnetii	42–84	IgG, IgM

Adapted from Blank M, Asherson R A, Cervera R, et al. Antiphospholipid syndrome infectious origin. J Clin Immunol 2004:24(1):12–23; with permission.

Antiphospholipid Antibodies in Leprosy

aCL isotypes IgG, IgM, and IgA are elevated in some leprosy patients [62]. The aCL may be B_2 GPI dependent, particularly in patients who have the multibacillary type of leprosy [63]. An association was found between the presence of aCL and certain dermatologic manifestations of leprosy, such as Raynaud's phenomenon, skin nodules, chronic skin ulcers, and urticarial rash [16]. Lucio's phenomenon is a rare manifestation of leprosy in which the histopathologic findings are related to microvascular thrombosis in the absence of inflammatory infiltration of the vessel walls. Levy and colleagues [64] demonstrated that this type of leprosy was associated with B_2 GPI dependence of aCL.

Antiphospholipid Antibodies in Streptococcal Infection

Streptococcal infections may be associated with increases in aCL, predominantly isotypes IgG in acute poststreptococcal glomerulonephritis and streptococcal impetigo without renal involvement [65]. Considerable controversy exists regarding acute rheumatic fever and rheumatic heart disease, with some investigators reporting raised aCL titers [66] and others not confirming these findings [67].

Antiphospholipid Antibodies in Leptospirosis

The prevalence of aPL during leptospiral infection is 23% for IgG and 10% for IgM and is not associated with thrombotic events [68]. These antibodies are predominant in patients who have severe infection. Tattevin and colleagues [69] reported a case of a 63-year-old man who had severe leptospirosis infection with considerable pulmonary hypertension (a feature of APS) and very high levels of aPL; he achieved complete resolution and normalization of aPL level with aggressive antibiotic therapy.

Antiphospholipid Antibodies in Coxiella Burnetii Infection

Q fever, caused by *Coxiella burnetii*, is associated with a high frequency of aCL positivity. In their study of 26 patients who had Q fever diagnosed by clinical and serologic criteria, Ordi-Ros and colleagues [70] reported a high incidence of IgM and IgG isotypes of aCL and that these antibodies can help diagnose Q fever presenting only as fever; antibodies to *Coxiella burnetii* and aCL are different antibodies and the aCL activity in patients who have Q fever is cofactor independent.

Antiphospholipid Antibodies in Mycoplasma Infection

Increased IgM and IgG aCL are detected in *Mycoplasma pneumoniae* infection. High titers were found in patients who had severe infections (needing hospitalization), in patients who had cold agglutinins, and in those who had extrapulmonary complications [71]. Cotter and colleagues [72] reported a patient who had severe *Mycoplasma pneumoniae* infection with transverse myelitis that improved with plasmapheresis. *Mycoplasma penetrans*, a rare bacterium, has been found so far only in HIV-infected persons [73]. Yanez and colleagues [74] reported on a 17-year-old non-HIV woman with *Mycoplasma penetrans* isolated from blood and throat who developed the clinical features of APS (hemolytic anemia, positive Coombs test, livedo reticularis, and paraparesis) and elevated aPL and LA titers. The patient clinically improved after intensive antibiotic therapy.

CATASTROPHIC ANTIPHOSPHOLIPID SYNDROME AND INFECTIONS

Catastrophic APS (CAPS), an unusual and potentially fatal subset of APS, was first described in 1992 [75]. As of 2004, 220 patients with this syndrome had been described and it comprises 1% of cases of APS [76]. It is characterized by evidence of the involvement of three or more organs, systems, or tissues, and the development of manifestations simultaneously or in less than a week, with confirmation by histopathology of small vessel occlusion in at least one organ or tissue and laboratory confirmation of the presence of aPL (LA or aCL) [77]. The disease is predominantly seen in women (70% of cases). Presentation of CAPS is often rapid and complex with involvement of renal (70%), pulmonary (65%), cerebral (55%), cardiac (50%), and gastrointestinal (44%) vessels. LA is detected in 79% of cases and aCL in high titers is seen in 86% of patients. Mortality is 47% and occurs from cardiac or respiratory failure or gastrointestinal involvement [78].

Several triggering factors can precipitate CAPS, including trauma, withdrawal of anticoagulation, carcinoma, and infections. Rojas-Rodriguez [79] reported infections to precede the appearance of CAPS; 35% to 40% of cases develop CAPS after infectious episodes [80], including respiratory (15%); cutaneous, including infected leg ulcers (8%); urinary tract (6%); gastrointestinal (1%); general sepsis (1%); and others (9%) [6]. More viral, as opposed to bacterial, infections act as trigger factors for CAPS [6]. It is suggested that antigens of *Salmonella* Typhi, such as lipopolysaccharides, may have immunologic and prothrombotic effects [81].

Most of the infectious agents may act as superantigens and, by way of a molecular mimicry phenomenon, lead to a disproportionate immune response by inducing nonpathogenic aPL and pathogenic anti–B_2 GPI antibodies. Therefore, it may be possible to prevent this devastating evolution if the infectious process is recognized promptly and treated aggressively.

SUMMARY

aPL with their protein cofactors are essential for the diagnosis of APS. aPL of different kinds are detected in many infections, although in low titers and without protein cofactors in most cases.

aPL found in APS can be differentiated from those found in infections by determining LA activity and anti–B_2 GPI antibodies. LA activity and anti–B_2 GPI are present in APS resulting in thrombotic manifestations but not in most cases of infection (nonthrombogenic aPL). However, in several infections (leprosy, parvovirus B_{19}, HIV, HCV, CMV), the aCL may be B_2 GPI dependent, resembling those found in autoimmune diseases; are clearly heterogenous and pathogenic; and may be accompanied by thrombotic manifestation.

Various infections are associated with the triggering of the potentially lethal subset of APS, CAPS. This situation requires prompt diagnosis and aggressive treatment of the infection to prevent severe complications.

Acknowledgment

The author sincerely appreciates the secretarial assistance given by Alicia M. Chavez and Cynthia Rodriguez in the preparation of this article.

References

[1] Asherson RA, Khamashta MA, Ordi-Ros J, et al. The primary antiphospholipid syndrome: major clinical and serological features. Medicine 1989;68:366–74.

[2] Wilson WA, Gharavi AE, Koike T, et al. International consensus statement on preliminary criteria for definite antiphospholipid syndrome. Report of an international workshop. Arthritis Rheum 1999;42:1309–11.

[3] Cervera R, Piette JC, Font J, et al. Antiphospholipid syndrome, clinical and immunologic manifestations and pattern of disease expression in a cohort of 1000 patients. Arthritis Rheum 2002;46:1019–27.

[4] Asherson RA, Cervera R. Primary, secondary and other varients of the antiphospholipid syndrome. Lupus 1994;3:293–8.

[5] Uthman IW, Gharavi AE. Viral infections and antiphospholipid antibodies. Semin Arthritis Rheum 2002;31(4):256–63.

[6] Asherson RA, Cervera R. Antiphospholipid antibodies and infections. Ann Rheum Dis 2003;62:388–93.

[7] Galli M, Comfurius P, Massen C, et al. Anticardiolipin antibodies directed not to cardiolipin but to plasma protein cofactor. Lancet 1990;335:1544–7.

[8] Hunt JE, Mc Neil HP, Morgan GI, et al. A phospholipid B—B_2 glycoprotein I complex in an antigen for cardiolipin antibodies occurring in autoimmune disease but not with infection. Lupus 1992;1:75–81.

[9] Fiallo P, Nunzi E, Cardo PP. B_2 glycoprotein 1 dependent anticardiolipin antibodies as risk factors for reactions in borderline leprosy patients. Int J Lepr Other Mycobact Dis 1998;66: 387–8.

[10] Loizou S, Cazabon JK, Walport MJ, et al. Similarities of specificity and cofactor dependence in serum antiphospholipid antibodies from patients with human parvo virus B_{19} infections and those with SLE. Arthritis Rheum 1997;40:103–8.

[11] Blank M, Asherson RA, Cervera R, et al. Antiphospholipid syndrome infectious origin. J Clin Immunol 2004;24(1):12–23.

[12] Albert LJ, Inman RD. Molecular mimicry and autoimmunity. N Engl J Med 1999;341: 2068–74.

[13] Blank M, Krauss I, Fridkin M, et al. Bacterial induction of autoantibodies to beta 2 glycoprotein I accounts for the infectious etiology of antiphospholipid syndrome. J Clin Invest 2002;109:797–804.

[14] Shoenfeld Y, Blank M, Lervra R, et al. Infectious origin of antiphospholipid syndrome. Ann Rheum Dis 2006;65:2–6.

[15] Dalekos GN, Zachou K, Liaskos C. The antiphospholipid syndrome and infection. Curr Rheumatol Rep 2001;3:277–85.

[16] Zandman-Goddard G, Blank M, Shoenfeld Y, et al. Antiphospholipid antibodies and infection-drugs. In: Asherson RA, Gervera R, Shoenfeld Y, editors. The antiphospholipid syndrome II—autoimmune thrombosis. Amsterdam (Netherlands): Elsevier; 2002. p. 343–58.

[17] Cervera R, Asherson RA, Acevedo MI, et al. Antiphospholipid syndrome associated with infection. Clinical and microbiological characteristics in 100 patients. Ann Rheum Dis 2004;63:1312–7.

[18] Cacoub P, Renou C, Rosenthal E, et al. Extrahepatic manifestations associated with hepatitis C virus infection. Medicine 2000;79:47–56.
[19] Leroy V, Arvieux J, Jacob MC, et al. Prevalence and significance of anticardiolipin, anti B_2 glycoprotein I and antithrombin antibodies in chronic hepatitis C. Br J Haematol 1998;101: 468–74.
[20] Prieto J, Yuste JR, Beloqui O, et al. Anticardiolipin antibodies in chronic hepatitis C: implication of hepatitis C virus as a cause of APS. Hepatology 1996;23:199–204.
[21] Sthoeger ZM, Fogel M, Smirov A, et al. Anticardiolipin autoantibodies in serum samples and cryoglobulins of patients with hepatitis C infection. Ann Rheum Dis 2000;59: 483–6.
[22] Ordi-Ros J, Villarreal J, Monegal F, et al. Anticardiolipin antibodies in patients with chronic hepatitis C virus infection: characterization in relation to antiphospholipid syndrome. Clin Diagn Lab Immunol 2000;7:241–4.
[23] Harada J, Fujisawa Y, Sakisaka S, et al. High prevalence of anticardiolipin antibodies in hepatitis C infection: lack of effects on thrombocytopenia and thrombotic complications. J Gastroenterol 2000;35:272–7.
[24] Mangia A, Margaglione M, Cascavilla I, et al. Anticardiolipin antibodies in patients with liver diseases. Am J Gastroenterol 1999;94:2983–7.
[25] Caloub P, Mosset L, Amoura Z, et al. Anticardiolipin, anti B_2 glycoprotein I, and antinucleosome antibodies in hepatitis C virus infection and mixed cryoglobulinemia. J Rheumatol 1997;24:139–44.
[26] Biron C, Andreani H, Blang P, et al. Prevalence of antiphospholipid antibodies in patients with chronic liver disease related to alcohol or hepatitis C: correlation with liver injury. J Lab Clin Med 1998;131:243–50.
[27] Gioradano P, Galli M, Del Vecchio GC, et al. Lupus anticoagulant, anticardiolipin antibodies and hepatitis C in thalassaemia. Br J Haematol 1998;102:903–6.
[28] Baid S, Pasgual M, William WW, et al. Renal thrombotic microangiopathy associated with anticardiolipin antibodies in hepatitis C positive renal allografts recipients. J Am Soc Nephrol 1999;10:146–53.
[29] Malnick SS, Abend Y, Euron E, et al. HCV hepatitis associated with anticardiolipin antibody and cerebrovascular accidents, response to interferon therapy. J Clin Gastroenterol 1997;24:40–2.
[30] Matsuda J, Saitoh N, Gotoh M, et al. High prevalence of anti-phospholipid antibodies and anti-thyroglobulin antibody in patients with hepatitis C virus infection treated with interferon-alpha. Am J Gastroenterol 1995;90:1138–41.
[31] Bloom EJ, Abrams DI, Rodgers G. Lupus anticoagulant in acquired immunodeficiency syndrome. JAMA 1986;258:491–3.
[32] Argov S, Shanttner Y, Burstein R, et al. Autoantibodies in male homosexuals and HIV infections. Immunol Lett 1991;30:31–6.
[33] De Larranga GF, Forastoero RR, Carreras LC, et al. Different types of antiphospholipid antibodies in AIDS: a comparison with syphilis and the antiphospholipid syndrome. Thromb Res 1999;95:19–25.
[34] Ordi J, Selua A, Monegal F, et al. Protein S and HIV infection. The role of anticardiolipin and anti-protein S antibodies. J Rheumatol 1993;8:1321–4.
[35] Petrovas C, Vlachoyiannopoulos PG, Kordossis T, et al. Antiphospholipid antibodies in HIV infection and SLE with or without anti-phospholipid syndrome: comparisons of phospholipid specificity, avidity and reactivity with B_2-GPI. J Autoimmun 1999;13: 347–55.
[36] Silvestris F, Frassanito MA, Cafforio P, et al. Antiphosphatidylserine antibodies in human immunodeficiency virus-I patients with evidence of T-cell apoptosis and mediate antibody-dependent cellular cytotoxicity. Blood 1996;87:5185–95.
[37] Abuaf N, Laperche S, Rajoely B, et al. Autoantibodies to phospholipids and to coagulation protein in AIDS. Thromb Haemost 1997;77:856–61.

[38] Brew BJ, Miller J. Human immunodeficiency virus type I related to transient neurological deficits. Am J Med 1996;101:257–61.
[39] Guerin J, Casey E, Feighery C, et al. Anti B_2 GPI antibody isotype and IgG subclass in antiphospholipid syndrome patients. Autoimmunity 1999;31:109–16.
[40] Coll J, Gutierrez-Cebollada J, Yazbeck H, et al. Anticardiolipin antibodies and acquired immunodeficiency syndrome: prognostic marker or association with HIV infection. Infection 1992;20:140–2.
[41] Falco M, Sorrenli A, Priori R, et al. Anticardiolipin antibodies in HIV infection are true antiphospholipids not associated with antiphospholipid syndrome. Ann Ital Med Int 1993;8:171–4.
[42] Becker DM, Saunder TJ, Wispelway B, et al. Case report venous thromboembolism in AIDS. Am J Med Sci 1992;42:327–8.
[43] Park KL, Marx JL, Lopez PF, et al. Noninfectious branch retinal vein occlusion in HIV positive patient. Retina 1997;17:162–4.
[44] Meyohas MC, Roullet E, Rouzioux C, et al. Central venous sinus thrombosis and dual primary infection with HIV and CMV. J Neurol Neurosurg Psychiatry 1998;52:1010–1.
[45] Carr A, Brown D, Cooper DA. Portal vein thrombosis in patients receiving indinavir, an HIV protease inhibitor. AIDS 1997;11:1657–8.
[46] Wang L, Molina CP, Rajaraman S. Case report: intestinal infarction due to vascular catastrophe in an HIV-infected patient. AIDS Read 2000;10:718–25.
[47] Leder AN, Flansbaum B, Zandman-Goddard G, et al. Antiphospholipid syndrome induced by HIV. Lupus 2001;10:370–4.
[48] Bosson JL, Fleury-Feuillade MI, Farah I, et al. Arterial and venous thromboembolic disease in an HIV positive patient. J Mal Vasc 1995;20:136–8.
[49] Thirumalai S, Kirshner HS. Anticardiolipin antibody and stroke in an HIV-positive patient. AIDS 1994;8:1019–20.
[50] Cappell MS, Simon T, Tiku M. Splenic infarction associated with anticardiolipin antibodies with AIDS. Dig Dis Sci 1993;38:1153–5.
[51] Belmonte MA, Garcia-Portales R, Domenech I, et al. Avascular necrosis of bone in human immunodeficiency virus infection and antiphospholipid antibodies. J Rheumatol 1993;20:1425–8.
[52] Jenkin RE, Peters BS, Pinching AJ. Thromboembolic disease in AIDS associated with cytomegalovirus disease. AIDS 1991;5:1540–2.
[53] Labarca JA, Rabaggliati RM, Radrigan FJ, et al. Antiphospholipid syndrome associated with CMV infection: case report and review. Clin Infect Dis 1997;25:1493–4.
[54] Uthman T, Tabbarah Z, Gharavi AE. Hughes syndrome associated cytomegalovirus infection. Lupus 1999;8:775–7.
[55] Smith KJ, Skelton HG, Yeafer J, et al. Cutaneous thrombosis in HIV-I positive patients and CMV viraemia. Arch Dermatol 1995;131:357–8.
[56] Mengarelli A, Minotti C, Palumbo G, et al. High levels of antiphospholipid antibodies with CMV infection in unrelated bone marrow and cord blood allogeneic stem cell transplantation. Br J Haematol 2000;108:126–31.
[57] Uthman T, Taher A, Khalil I. Hughes syndrome associated with varicella infection. Rheumatol Int 2001;20:167–8.
[58] Manco-Johnson MJ, Nuss R, Key N, et al. Lupus anticoagulant and protein S deficiency in children with postvaricella purpura fulminans or thrombosis. J Pediatr 1996;128:319–23.
[59] Faghiri Z, Wilson WA, Taheri J, et al. Antibodies to cardiolipin and B_2 glycoprotein I in HTLV-I associated myelopathy/tropical spastic paraparesis. Lupus 1999;8:210–4.
[60] Sorice M, Pittoni V, Griggi T, et al. Specificity of anti phospholipids antibodies in infectious mononucleosis: are all for anti-cofactor protein antibodies. Clin Exp immunol 2000;120:301–6.
[61] Yamazaki M, Asakura H, Kawamura Y, et al. Transient lupus anticoagulant induced by Epstein-Barr virus infection. Blood Coagul Fibrinolysis 1991;2:771–4.

[62] de Larranga GF, Forasttero RR, Martinuzzo ME, et al. High prevalence of antiphospholipid antibodies in leprosy-evaluation of antigen reactivity. Lupus 2000;9:594–600.
[63] Fiallo P, Travaglino C, Nunzi E, et al. B$_2$ glycoprotein dependence of anticardiolipin antibodies in multibacillary leprosy patients. Lepr Rev 1998;69:376–81.
[64] Levy RA, Pierangeli SA, Espinola RG, et al. Antiphospholipid beta-2 glycoprotein I dependency assay to determine antibody pathogenicity. Arthritis Rheum 2000;43(Suppl):1476.
[65] Ardiles L, Ramirez P, Moya P, et al. Anticardiolipin antibodies in acute poststreptococcal glomerulonephritis and streptococcal impetigo. Nephron 1999;83:47–52.
[66] Figueroa F, Berrios X, Gutierrez M, et al. Anticardiolipin antibodies in acute rheumatic fever. J Rheumatol 1992;19:1175–80.
[67] Ilarraza H, Marquez MF, Alcocer A, et al. Anticardiolipin antibodies are not associated with rheumatic heart disease. Lupus 2001;10:873–5.
[68] Rugman FP, Pinn G, Palmer G, et al. Anticardiolipin antibodies in leptospirosis. J Clin Pathol 1991;44:517–9.
[69] Tattevin P, Dupeux S, Hoff J, et al. Leptospirosis and the antiphospholipid syndrome. Am J Med 2003;114:164.
[70] Ordi-Ros J, Selva-O'Callaghan A, Monegal-Ferran F, et al. Prevalence, significance and specificity of antibodies to phospholipids in Q fever. Clin Infect Dis 1994;18:213–8.
[71] Snowden N, Wilson PB, Longson M, et al. Antiphospholipid antibodies and Mycoplasma pneumoniae infection. Postgrad Med J 1990;66:356–62.
[72] Cotter FE, Bainbridge D, Newland AC, et al. Neurological deficit associated with Mycoplasma pneumoniae reversed by plasma exchange. Br Med J 1983;286:22.
[73] Grau O, Slizewicz B, Tuppin P, et al. Association of Mycoplasma penetrans with immunodeficiency virus infection. J Infect Dis 1995;172:672–81.
[74] Yanez A, Codillo L, Neyrolles O, et al. Mycoplasma penetrans bacteremia and primary antiphospholipid syndrome. Emerg Infect Dis 1999;5(1):1–6.
[75] Asherson RA. The catastrophic antiphospholipid syndrome. J Rheumatol 1992;19:508–12.
[76] Asherson RA. The catastrophic antiphospholipid syndrome registry project group. Lupus 2003;12:530–6.
[77] Cervera R, Gomez-Puerta JA, Cucho M, et al. Catastrophic antiphospholipid syndrome: analysis of international consensus statement on preliminary classification criteria for CAPS using CAPS registry. Ann Rheum Dis 2003;62(Suppl):84.
[78] Michael-Belmont H. Catastrophic antiphospholipid syndrome. In: Asherson RA, Cervera R, Shoenfield Y, editors. The antiphospholipid syndrome II-autoimmune thrombosis. Amsterdam (Netherlands): Elsevier; 2002. p. 171–80.
[79] Rojas-Rodriguez J, Garcia-Carrasco M, Ramos-Casal M, et al. Catastrophic antiphospholipid syndrome: clinical description and triggering factors in 8 patients. J Rheumatol 1999;26:238–40.
[80] Asherson RA, Cervera R, Piette JC, et al. Catastrophic antiphospholipid syndrome: clues to the pathogenesis from a series of 80 patients. Medicine 2001;80:355–77.
[81] Hayem G, Kassis N, Nicaise P, et al. Systemic lupus erythematosus-associated catastrophic antiphospholipid syndrome occurring after typhoid fever: a possible role of salmonella lipopolysaccharide in the occurrence of diffuse vasculopathy-coagulopathy. Arthritis Rheum 1999;42:1056–65.

Treatment Options for Patients Who Have Antiphospholipid Syndromes

Rodger L. Bick, MD, PhD, FACP[a],*,
William F. Baker, MD, FACP[b,c,d]

[a]10455 North Central Expressway, Suite 109-320, Dallas, TX 75231, USA
[b]David Geffen School of Medicine Center for Health Sciences University of California, Los Angeles, Los Angeles, CA, USA
[c]Thrombosis, Hemostasis and Special Hematology Clinic, Kern Medical Center, Bakersfield, CA, USA
[d]California Clinical Thrombosis Center, 9330 Stockdale Highway, Suite 300, Bakersfield, CA 93211, USA

The antiphospholipid thrombosis syndrome, associated with anticardiolipin (aCL) or subgroup antibodies (Box 1), can be divided into one of six subgroups:

- Type I syndrome comprises patients with deep venous thrombosis (DVT) and pulmonary embolism (PE).
- Type II syndrome comprises patients with coronary artery or peripheral arterial (including aorta and carotid artery) thrombosis.
- Type III syndrome comprises patients with retinal or cerebrovascular (intracranial) thrombosis.
- Type IV patients are those with admixtures of the first three types. Type IV patients are uncommon, with most patients fitting into one of the first three types.
- Type V patients are those with recurrent miscarriage syndrome.
- Type VI patients are those harboring antiphospholipid syndromes (APSs) without any (as yet) clinical expression, including thrombosis.

There is little overlap (about 10% or less) between these subtypes, and patients usually conveniently fit into only one of these clinical types. The types of antiphospholipid and thrombosis syndromes associated with aCL antibodies are summarized in Box 2 [1–3]. Although there appears to be no correlation with the type, or titer, of aCL antibody and type of syndrome (I–VI), the subclassification of thrombosis and aCL antibody patients into these groups is important from the therapy standpoint [1–3]. Type I patients are best managed by use of long-term fixed-dose low molecular weight heparin (LMWH) or

*Corresponding author. E-mail address: rbick@thrombosis.com (R.L. Bick).

> **Box 1: Antiphospholipid syndrome antibodies**
>
> Lupus anticoagulant
> Beta-2-glycoprotein-1 (IgG, IgA, IgM)
> Anticardiolipin antibodies (IgG, IgA, IgM)
> - Antiphosphatidylserine (IgG, IgA, IgM)
> - Antiphosphatidylinositol (IgG, IgA, IgM)
> - Antiphosphatidylcholine (IgG, IgA, IgM)
> - Antiphosphatidic acid (IgG, IgA, IgM)
> - Antiphosphatidylethanolamine (IgG, IgA, IgM)
> - Antiphosphatidic acid (IgG, IgA, IgM)
> - Antiphosphatidylglycerol (IgG, IgA, IgM)
> - Anti-annexin-V antibody (IgG, IgA, IgM)

fixed-dose subcutaneous unfractionated heparin (UFH) therapy. If the patient remains thrombus free for 6 to 12 months, or if osteoporosis becomes a consideration, long-term clopidogrel may eventually be substituted for the heparin/LMWH. Type II patients are also best managed by long-term fixed-dose LMWH (about 5000 units/24 hours) or fixed-dose subcutaneous UFH therapy (usually 5000 units every 12 hours) and, after long-term stability, clopidogrel may be an alternative. Type III patients—those with cerebrovascular disease or retinal vascular disease—should be treated with fixed-dose long-term LMWH plus clopidogrel for intracranial/cerebral vessel thrombosis/transient ischemic attack (TIA); long-term stability can usually be achieved by stopping the heparin/LMWH and continuing clopidogrel. Clopidogrel (at 75 mg/day) is usually effective for retinal vascular thrombosis, and if failure occurs, LMWH may be added to the clopidogrel therapy. Therapy of type IV depends on types and sites of thrombosis present [1–3]. Patients with type V, recurrent miscarriage syndrome, are best treated with preconception initiation of low-dose aspirin (ASA) at 81 mg/day as soon as the diagnosis is made and then started on fixed, low-dose porcine mucosal heparin (5000 units, subcutaneously every 12 hours) or LMWH at 5000 units/day immediately postconception, with both drugs—a heparin compound and ASA—being used to term delivery [4]. Patients with type V syndrome are usually encouraged to stop the heparin following delivery (depending on the individual clinical situation) but to continue on long-term, low-dose ASA indefinitely. The decision to continue ASA after delivery in these patients is empiric, but might ward off other minor thrombotic manifestations of APS. There are no guidelines available to know how to best treat these patients following delivery, as most (<10%) will not develop a nonplacental thrombosis.

Obviously, patients with thrombosis and aCL antibodies require long-term antithrombotic therapy, and treatment should be stopped only if the aCL antibody is persistently absent for at least 6 months before considering cessation of antithrombotic therapy [1–3]. After persistent absence of the

> **Box 2: Types of antiphospholipid thrombosis syndromes**
>
> *Type I syndrome*
> - Deep venous thrombosis with or without pulmonary embolus
>
> *Type II syndrome*
> - Coronary artery thrombosis
> - Peripheral artery thrombosis
> - Aortic thrombosis
> - Carotid artery thrombosis
>
> *Type III syndrome*
> - Retinal artery thrombosis
> - Retinal vein thrombosis
> - Cerebrovascular thrombosis
> - TIAs
>
> *Type IV syndrome*
> - Mixtures of types I, II, and III; type IV patients are rare
>
> *Type V (fetal wastage) syndrome*
> - Placental vascular thrombosis
> - Fetal wastage common in first trimester
> - Fetal wastage can occur in second and third trimesters; maternal thrombocytopenia (uncommon)
>
> *Type VI syndrome*
> - Antiphospholipid antibody with no apparent clinical manifestations

antiphospholipid (aPL) antibody for at least 6 months, the clinician should assess and usually discuss the risks and benefits of continuing antithrombotic therapy and encourage patients to take one low-dose ASA (81 mg/day) or long-term clopidogrel (depending on the seriousness of the initial thrombotic event or events), in hopes the antibody and thrombosis will not return. Obviously, patients with APS who are going to be on long-term, fixed low-dose UFH or LMWH therapy should have initial bone density studies and should be cautioned about heparin-induced thrombocytopenia, mild alopecia, mild allergic reactions, skin reactions, osteoporosis, benign transaminasemia (seen in about 5% treated with UFH and in about 10% treated with LMWH), and the development of benign eosinophilia [5,6]. Patients should be monitored with weekly heparin levels (anti-Xa method) and complete blood counts/platelet counts for the first month of therapy and monthly thereafter; this also applies to patients with type V syndrome [4]. Box 3 outlines suggested antithrombotic therapy regimens, based on type of anticardiolipin thrombosis

> **Box 3: Recommended antithrombotic regimens for syndromes of thrombosis associated with antiphospholipid antibodies**
>
> *Type I syndrome*
> - Acute treatment with heparin/LMWH followed by long-term self-administration of subcutaneous porcine heparin/LMWH clopidogrel (long-term if stable)
>
> *Type II syndrome*
> - Acute treatment with heparin/LMWH followed by long-term self-administration of subcutaneous porcine heparin/LMWH clopidogrel (long-term if stable)
>
> *Type III syndrome*
> - Cerebrovascular
> - Long-term (clopidogrel) plus long-term self-administration of subcutaneous porcine heparin/LMWH
> - Retinal
> - Clopidogrel; if failure, add long-term self-administration of subcutaneous porcine heparin/LMWH
>
> *Type IV syndrome*
> - Therapy depends on types and sites of thrombosis, as per preceding recommendations
>
> *Type V (fetal wastage) syndrome*
> - Low-dose aspirin (81 mg/day) before conception and add fixed, low-dose porcine heparin at 5000 units every 12 hours or dalteparin (Fragmin) at 5000 units/day immediately after conception
>
> *Type VI syndrome*
> - No clear indications for antithrombotic therapy; antithrombotic therapy should not be stopped unless the antibodies have been absent for the preceding 6 months

syndrome. Many patients who have thrombosis and aPL antibodies fail warfarin therapy. The clinician always should suspect and search for aPL antibodies when evaluating a patient who has warfarin failure. Therapeutic anticoagulation with warfarin to a target INR of 2–3 for patients who have type I and type II APS has been studied extensively and recommended. For venous thrombosis, full anticoagulation with adjusted dose UFH or therapeutic dose LMWH for at least 6–12 months is recommended. Concern regarding warfarin failure has led the authors to recommend the use of a heparin drug rather then warfarin for long-term therapy. Clinical trial data are insufficient to determine clearly which therapy is superior.

CLINICAL PRESENTATIONS

It is becoming increasingly clear with increased experience in using the anticardiolipin assay in clinical practice that primary APSs are much more common than suspected. Diagnostic evaluation of the patient to determine the etiology of a wide variety of thrombotic problems must now include assays for aCL antibodies, lupus anticoagulants, and, when indicated, subgroups. Although it is appropriate to suspect aPL antibodies in virtually any clinical problem complicated by thrombosis, certain presentations are stronger indicators than others.

In patients with type I disease, a strong index of suspicion is appropriate, particularly in individuals with DVT unaccompanied by another potential risk factor (eg, exogenous estrogen administration, surgery, prolonged immobility, malignancy, or another hypercoagulable state). Likewise, patients may present with recurrent DVT with or without a significant clinical risk factor. As is frequently observed in clinical practice, patients may be referred for evaluation only after a second episode of thrombosis. The initial thrombotic event may have appeared to result from a recognizable predisposing problem, only later proven to be present concomitantly with aCL antibodies. Although the severity or location (iliofemoral, popliteal calf vein, or other sites) of thrombosis or the presence of pulmonary embolization does not correlate with the presence of aCL antibodies, recurrent thromboembolic events or multiple sites of thrombosis should strongly suggest an aPL antibody. Another common presentation is a patient referred because of failure (rethrombosis) while on warfarin therapy. Failure to apparently adequate doses of warfarin should immediately alert the physician to strongly consider APS.

Patients with type II disease frequently present with catastrophic illness. A history of myocardial infarction at a young age, recurrent myocardial infarction, early graft occlusion following coronary artery bypass graft surgery, and early re-occlusion following post-transluminal angioplasty is typical [7]. Aorta, subclavian, mesenteric, femoral, or other large-vessel thrombosis may present with complete occlusion and acute symptoms of ischemia and threatened limb loss. Emergent diagnosis and appropriate therapy may decrease unnecessary morbidity and be life-saving.

Type III patients may be referred for a variety of problems. Acute loss or distortion of vision may lead to ophthalmologic confirmation of retinal arterial or venous thrombosis. Focal neurologic symptoms may suggest the presence of cerebrovascular thrombosis resulting in symptoms of stroke or TIA. Alternatively, multiple infarct dementia may present more gradually, without clearly defined acute ischemic events. Early diagnosis is critical in type III patients, as failure to treat may result in irreversible central nervous system or retinal injury.

Type IV patients, having a mixture of the aforementioned types, are extremely rare and comprise only about 1% of patients with anticardiolipin thrombosis syndrome. A strong index of suspicion is required for the diagnosis, and therapy must be individualized depending on the particular combination of thromboses.

Type V patients are usually those with one or more spontaneous miscarriages and are most often referred by the obstetrician or high-risk reproductive experts. Most women relate a history of spontaneous miscarriage in the first trimester (most commonly the 6th–12th week), but some also spontaneously miscarry in the second and third trimesters.

PREVALENCE OF THE ANTIPHOSPHOLIPID THROMBOSIS SYNDROME

Unfortunately, little information is available on prevalence of aPL antibodies, especially in asymptomatic individuals. Additionally, nothing is known about the potential propensity to develop thrombosis or other clinical manifestations when seemingly healthy individuals are found to harbor these antibodies. Two recent studies have addressed this issue. The first such study was the Montpellier Antiphospholipid study [8], wherein 1014 patients (488 males, 526 females) admitted to a general internal medicine department for a variety of reasons were assessed for IgG, IgA, and IgM aCL antibodies. Lupus anticoagulant assays were not performed. Of the patients tested, 72 (7.1%) were positive for at least one idiotype. When assessing these 72 patients, 20 (28%) were determined to have clinical manifestations of APS. Fifty-two patients, when questioned, had not yet demonstrated any manifestations of APL-T syndrome, suggesting a false-positive incidence of 5.1%. However, long-term follow-up of the thus far asymptomatic patients has not occurred, and a follow-up report of the Montpellier Antiphospholipid study will be awaited with interest. In another recent study [9], 552 healthy blood donors were screened for study; IgG and IgM idiotypes and lupus anticoagulant were assessed. It was found that 6.5% (28 donors) of the population harbored IgG, 9.4% (38 donors) of the population harbored IgM aCL antibodies, and 5 donors had both idiotypes. No donor was positive for lupus anticoagulant. The donors were followed for 12 months; during the follow-up time, no aCL-positive patient developed a thrombotic event. However, 9 aCL-positive donors had a positive family history for thrombosis and 3 of the aCL-positive donors had a history of unexplained miscarriage.

In a patient harboring aPL antibodies and no symptoms, there is no clear evidence that any antithrombotic treatment is needed.

In a survey of 100 consecutive patients presenting with DVT or PE, 24% of patients were found to have aPL antibodies [10]. It is suggested that aPL antibodies are common in patients presenting with unexplained DVT or PE, and certainly any patient presenting with unexplained DVT or PE should be evaluated for presence of aPL antibodies.

General treatment programs have been outlined in this section. These are primarily developed from the present authors' clinical experience. For additional or alternate treatment strategies and recommendations, the reader is encouraged to see other articles in this issue.

International preliminary catastrophic antiphospholipid syndrome (CAPS) classification criteria and treatment guidelines were proposed by the 2002 International Taormina Consensus Statement on Classification and Treatment of CAPS [11]. Criteria for diagnosis include the involvement of three or more organs, systems, and/or tissues [11].

The approach to treatment has included a variety of modalities, including anticoagulation, glutocorticoids, plasmapheresis, cyclophosphamide, intravenous gammaglobulins, and splenectomy. Most patients, however, received a combination of nonsurgical therapies. In spite of combination therapy (most nonsurgical), death still occurred in 25 of the 50 (50%) patients reported by Asherson and colleagues [12]. The current rationale for the recommended therapy of combined anticoagulation, steroids, and plasmapheresis or intravenous gammaglobulins is derived from the reported survival rate of 70% in patients so treated [11]. The most successful approach is similar to that used in treatment of patients with thrombotic thrombocytopenic purpura and hemolytic uremic syndrome. The fibrinolytic agents streptokinase and urokinase have also been used [13,14]. There is, however, no large series comparing various therapies and combinations that can be relied on to provide firm recommendations [2].

Venous Thrombosis

Venous thrombosis typically presents with DVT in the lower extremities, observed in 29% to 55% of cases over a follow-up period of less than 6 years [7,8], [10]. As with all cases of venous thromboembolism (VTE), more than half of the patients with symptomatic DVT have asymptomatic PE [15]. When patients present with symptoms typical of PE, at least half will not exhibit clinical manifestations of DVT [16,17]. There is not a particular clinical pattern of venous thrombosis that suggests that the patient may have underlying aPL antibodies. Unusual sites of thrombosis have included venous thrombosis of the upper extremities, intracranial veins, inferior and superior vena cava, hepatic veins (Budd Chiari syndrome), portal vein, renal vein, and retinal vein [18–20]. Thrombosis of the cerebral veins may present with acute cerebral infarction [21]. The superficial and deep cerebral venous system may be extensively involved. Onset of cerebral venous thrombosis due to aPL antibodies typically presents at a younger age and in a more extensive pattern than in other patients. Thrombosis of the superior saggital sinus has also been reported. In one series of 40 patients with cerebral venous thrombosis, 3 had aPL antibodies and 2 of these 3 also had Factor V Leiden mutation [22].

In the setting of idiopathic VTE, laboratory assessment is recommended to search for the presence of underlying thrombophilia [15]. Supporting this is the series of 100 consecutive patients with idiopathic DVT or PE in which 24% were found to have aPL antibodies [23]. Testing for aPL antibodies is strongly recommend because of the high frequency with which APS is diagnosed [6]. Even in patients with a family history of venous thrombosis, which suggests an underlying inherited thrombophilic disorder, testing for aPL antibodies is indicated, as many patients with one thrombophilic disorder also have another. The clinical manifestations of VTE are the same, whether aPL antibodies are present or not. Subsequent to a first episode of VTE, the risk for future venous thrombosis increases significantly. In patients with APS, the risk doubles to at least a 30% risk of recurrence, without antithrombotic therapy.

Arterial Thrombosis

Arterial thromboses are less common than venous thrombosis [7,8], and occur in a variety of settings in patient with primary APS. Of the 1000 patients in the Euro-Phospholipid Trial, 13.1% presented with stroke, 7% with TIA, and 2.8%

with acute myocardial infarction [24]. Patients with arterial thrombosis most commonly present with TIA or stroke (50%) or myocardial infarction (23%) [7,24,25]. These relatively common arterial occlusive events most suggest APS when they occur in individuals without readily identified risk factors for atherosclerosis. This population primarily includes individuals under age 60, without classic risk factors for atherosclerosis (family history, cigarette smoking, hyperlipidemia, hypertension, diabetes mellitus) [19,26]. The presence of aCL antibody is considered to be a risk factor for first stroke [23]. Arterial thrombosis in patients with APS may also involve other large and small vessels, somewhat unusual for other thrombophilic disorders or atherosclerotic occlusive disease. These include thrombosis of brachial and subclavian arteries, axillary artery (aortic arch syndrome), aorta, iliac, femoral, renal, mesenteric, retinal, and other peripheral arteries [2,7]. Clinical manifestations, of course, depend on the caliber and location of the affected artery.

References

[1] Bick RL. Antiphospholipid thrombosis syndromes: etiology, pathophysiology, diagnosis and management. Int J Hematol 1997;65:193–213.

[2] Bick RL. The antiphospholipid thrombosis syndromes: a common multidisciplinary medical problem. J Clin Appl Thromb Hemost 1997;3:270–83.

[3] Bick RL. Hereditary and acquired thrombophilia. Clin Appl Thromb Hemost 2006;12:125–35.

[4] Bick RL. Recurrent miscarriage syndrome and Infertility caused by blood coagulation protein / platelet defects. Chapter 2. In: Bick RL, Frenkel E, Baker W, editors. Hematological complications in obstetrics, pregnancy and gynecology. Cambridge (UK): Cambridge University Press; 2006. p. 55–74.

[5] Walenga JM, Bick RL. Heparin-induced thrombocytopenia, paradoxical thromboembolism and other side effects of heparin therapy. Med Clin North Am 1998;82(3):635–58.

[6] Girolami B, Prandoni P, Rossi L, et al. Transaminase elevation in patients treated with unfractionated heparin or low molecular weight heparin for venous thromboembolism. Clin Appl Thromb Hemost 1998;4:126–8.

[7] Bick RL. Antiphospholipid thrombosis syndromes. Hematol Oncol Clin North Am 2003;17:115–47.

[8] Schved JF, Dupuy-Fons C, Biron C. A prespective epidemiological study on the occurrence of antiphospholipid antibody: the Montpellier Antiphospholipiod (MAP) Study. Haemostasis 1994;24:175–82.

[9] Vila P, Hernandez MC, Lopez-Fernandez MF. Prevalence, follow-up and clinical significance of the anticardiolipin antibodies in normal subjects. Thromb Haemost 1994;72:209–13.

[10] Bick RL, Baker WF. Deep vein thrombosis: prevalence of etiologic factors and results of management in 100 consecutive patients. Semin Thromb Hemost 1992;18:267–74.

[11] Asherson RA, Cervera R, de Groot PG, et al. Catastrophic and antiphospholipid syndrome: international consensus statement on classification criteria and treatment guidelines. Lupus 2003;12(7):530–4.

[12] Asherson RA, Cervera R, Piette JC, et al. Catastrophic antiphospholipid syndrome. Clinical and laboratory features of 50 patients. Medicine (Baltimore) 1998;77(3):195–207.

[13] Harris EN, Gharavi A, Hegde U, et al. Anticardiolipin antibodies in autoimmune thrombocytopenic purpura. Br J Haematol 1985;59(2):231–4.

[14] Matsuda J, Sanaka T, Gonichi K, et al. Occurence of thrombotic thrombocytopenic purpura in a systemic lupus patient with antiphospholipid antibodies in association with a decreased activity of von Willebrand-factor cleaving protease. Lupus 2002;11:463–4.

[15] Schulman S, Svenungsson E, Granqvist S, et al. Anticardolipin antibodies predict early recurrence of thromboembolism and death among patients with venous thromboembolism following anticoagulant therapy. Am J Med 1998;104:332–8.
[16] Khamashta M, Cuadrado M, Mujic F, et al. The management of thrombosis in the antiphospholipid-antibody syndrome. N Engl J Med 1995;332:993–7.
[17] Nzerue C, Hewan-Lowe K, Pierangeli S, et al. "Black swan in the kidney:" renal involvement in the antiphospholipid antibody syndrome. Kidney Int 2002;62:733–44.
[18] Dunn J, Noorily S, Petri M, et al. Antiphospholipid antibodies and retinal vascular disease. Lupus 1996;5:313–22.
[19] Nochy D, Daugas E, Droz D, et al. The intrarenal vascular lesions associated with primary antiphospholipid syndrome. J Am Soc Nephrol 1999;10(3):507–18.
[20] Carhuapoma J, Mitsias P, Levine SR. Cerebral venous thrombosis and anticardiolipin antibodies. Stroke 1997;28:2363–9.
[21] Deschiens M, Conrad J, Horellou M, et al. Coagulation studies, factor V Leiden, and anticardiolipin antibodies in 40 cases of cerebral venous thrombosis. Stroke 1996;27:1724–9.
[22] Provenzale JM. Anatomic distribution of venous thrombosis in patients with antiphospholipid antibody: image findings. AJR 1995;165:365–8.
[23] Bick R, baker W. Antiphospholipid syndrome and thrombosis. Semin Thromb Hemost 1999;25:333.
[24] Group TAAiSSA. Anticardiolipin antibodies are an independent risk factor for ischemic stroke. Neurology 1993;43:2069–73.
[25] Group TAAiSSA. Anticardiolipin antibodies and the risk of recurrent thrombo-occlusive events and death. Neurology 1997;48:91.
[26] Cervera R, Piette JC, Font J, et al. Antiphospholipid syndrome: clinical and immunologic manifestations and patterns of disease expression in a cohort of 1,000 patients. Arthritis Rheum 2002;46:1019–27.

HEMATOLOGY/ONCOLOGY CLINICS OF NORTH AMERICA

Controversies and Unresolved Issues in Antiphospholipid Syndrome Pathogenesis and Management

William F. Baker, Jr, MD, FACP[a,b,c,]*,
Rodger L. Bick, MD, PhD, FACP[d], Jawed Fareed, PhD, FAHA[e,f]

[a]David Geffen School of Medicine, Center for Health Sciences, University of California, Los Angeles, Los Angeles, CA, USA
[b]California Clinical Thrombosis Center, 9330 Stockdale Highway, Suite 300, Bakersfield, CA 93311, USA
[c]Thrombosis, Hemostasis and Special Hamatology Clinic, Kern Medical Center, Bakersfield, CA 93305, USA
[d]10455 North Central Expressway, Suite 109-320, Dallas, TX 75231, USA
[e]Department of Pathology and Pharmacology, Loyola University Chicago, 2160 S. First Avenue, Maywood, IL 60153, USA
[f]Department of Cardiovascular Surgery, Loyola University Chicago, 2160 S. First Avenue, Maywood, IL 60153, USA

In 1906, antiphospholipid antibodies (aPL) were first detected in patients who had syphilis as a complement fixing antibody that reacted with extracts from bovine hearts. In 1941, the antigen was identified as the mitochondrial phospholipid, cardiolipin [1]. The Venereal Disease Research Laboratory (VDRL) test for syphilis was based on this anticardiolipin (aCL). As population screening proceeded, it was recognized in the 1950s that many patients with systemic lupus erythematosus, but without clinical or confirmatory laboratory tests for syphilis, had a false-positive VDRL test [2,3]. Initially, false-positive VDRL tests in patients with systemic lupus erythematosus were found to be associated with prolongation of in vitro measures of coagulation. This phenomenon was given the term "lupus anticoagulant" [4]. Although initial reports associated lupus anticoagulant with hemorrhage, it was subsequently discovered that bleeding only occurred in patients who had in vivo hypo-prothrombinemia and significant thrombocytopenia or thrombasthenia [5]. The association between lupus anticoagulant, circulating anticoagulants, thromboembolism, and pregnancy loss was subsequently reported in the 1960s [6]. In 1983, Harris and associates [7] developed a solid phase immunoassay for aCL antibodies and, in 1985, the association with thrombosis was confirmed and the term

*Corresponding author. E-mail address: wbaker@thrombosiscenter.com (W.F. Baker, Jr).

antiphospholipid syndrome (APS) was coined [8]. Continuing investigation in the 1990s demonstrated that the plasma phospholipid-binding protein beta-2-glycoprotein (B-2-GP I) was necessary to bind to cardiolipin [9,10]. This requirement was not found to be present in syphilis or in patients with infections [11]. It was shown that antibodies are formed not only to cardiolipin bound to B-2-GP I complexed with phospholipid but also to B-2-GP I directly [9,12]. Investigation into the pathobiology of APS has also led to the identification anti–annexin V antibodies [13], anti-prothrombin antibodies, and autoantibodies to the antiphospholipid subtypes (phosphatidylserine, phosphatidylethanolamine, phosphatidylglycerol, phosphatidylinositol, phosphatidylcholine, and phosphatidic acid) [4,14].

The presence of autoantibodies to various phospholipids and phospholipid-binding proteins has been identified in patients with large-vessel arterial and venous thrombosis, microvascular thrombosis, placental thrombosis, and a variety of other manifestations. The consequences of these vascular occlusions are found to affect virtually every organ and tissue.

While much is understood concerning the clinical features of patients with APS, many questions and controversial issues remain. There are many unanswered questions regarding pathogenesis. The proper designation of patients with "definite" APS and the correct categorization of patients by both laboratory and clinical features are matters of ongoing debate. Recent proposals have identified new subsets of patients who have many typical features of APS but either do not fit the criteria for a "definite" diagnosis [15] or who have initially negative laboratory tests for aPL [16]. The approach to diagnosis is also in question. Decisions about which laboratory test to order on which patient and which laboratory test to order when are based on expert opinion, rather than controlled trials. While many publications deal with treatment of APS, many issues remain unresolved. While many guidelines are offered, few are backed by data from strong clinical trials. This article summarizes the clinical questions remaining to be answered (Box 1) and debates concerning pathogenesis (Box 2), diagnosis (Box 3), and management (Box 4).

PATHOGENESIS

The early laboratory investigations of the serum of patients with syphilis triggered a sequence of discoveries leading to much of the current understanding of APS. Case reports and a small series of patients with biologically false-positive tests for syphilis and later lupus anticoagulant and aCL antibodies were simply reports of clinical associations with laboratory results. Intensive investigation has subsequently attempted to precisely determine the molecular biology involved with both the laboratory phenomena and the clinical manifestations (see Box 2).

Debate has centered on whether aPL directly cause thrombosis, are a consequence of thrombosis, or are simply an epiphenomenon. aPL may also function simply as a "second hit," both causing thrombosis and representing the result of antibody-mediated cellular injury [28]. Exposed anionic phospholipids may lead to immunological recognition and the generation of additional antibodies

> **Box 1: APS: questions to be answered**
>
> Is the presence of aPL a primary risk factor for thrombosis?
>
> Is the presence of aPL a primary risk factor for atherosclerosis?
>
> Is the presence of aPL a primary risk factor for pregnancy loss?
>
> Does the presence of asymptomatic aPL require measures to prevent a first thrombotic event? Does the benefit of such therapy outweigh the potential risks?
>
> Is aPL associated with recurrent arterial or venous thrombosis or recurrent pregnancy loss?
>
> Is acute management for thrombosis in the presence of aPL different from such management in the absence of aPL?
>
> Do aPL play a role in the development of cardioembolic strokes?
>
> What is optimal management to prevent recurrent arterial and venous thrombosis in patients with APS?
>
> If aPL become negative in a patient with a prior thrombotic event, should therapy be altered?
>
> What is optimal type, duration, and intensity of antithrombotic therapy?
>
> What are the best tests to order when APS is suspected?
>
> How should patients with clinical manifestations of APS but negative laboratory tests for aPL be managed?
>
> How should patients be managed who have clinical features of APS ("pre-APS" and microangiopathic phospholipid syndromes) and who test positive for aPL, but who do not fit the 2006 International Consensus criteria for APS?

[38]. Evidence has increasingly accumulated that the aPL are, in fact, directly responsible for vascular thrombosis [38].

A variety of experimental findings point to possible triggering events for the formation of autoantibodies to phospholipid and B-2-GP I [18,39]. These mechanisms have included:

- Overproduction of natural antibodies [17]
- Molecular mimicry resulting from infection [18]
- Exposure of phospholipids during platelet activation and cellular apoptosis (normally intracellular anionic phospholipids redistributed to the extracellular compartment) [19]
- Cardiolipin peroxidation [20]
- Platelet activation with or without antiplatelet antibodies [21]
- Genetic predisposition [22]

It is likely that a combination of pathologic interactions is necessary for the development of aPL. Once aPL are present, a complex cycle may develop such that apoptosis may elicit the formation of aPL but also then induce additional apoptosis. Apoptosis may then cause oxidative cellular injury, which also induces apoptosis. Pathologic activation of platelets and injury to endothelial

> **Box 2: Unresolved issues in pathogenesis**
>
> *Triggers to the development of aPL*
> Overproduction of natural antibodies [17]
> Molecular mimicry resulting from infection [18]
> Exposure of phospholipids during platelet activation and cellular apoptosis (normally intracellular anionic phospholipids redistributed to the extracellular compartment) [19]
> Cardiolipin peroxidation [20]
> Platelet activation with or without antiplatelet antibodies [21]
> Genetic predisposition [22]
>
> *Molecular mechanisms leading to thrombosis*
> Inhibition of endothelial cell prostacyclin production [23]
> Procoagulant effect on platelets [21]
> Impairment of fibrinolysis [24]
> Interference with the thrombomodulin–protein S–protein C pathway [25]
> Induction of procoagulant activity on endothelial cells and/or monocytes [26]
> Disruption of the annexin V cellular shield [13]
> Abnormal cytotrophoblast expression of adhesion molecules in pregnancy [27]
>
> *Is a "second hit" necessary for clinical thrombosis?* [28]

cells by aPL may result in exposure of anionic phospholipids and further stimulate the formation of aPL [40].

Proposed mechanisms of aPL-mediated thrombosis have included:

   Inhibition of endothelial cell prostacyclin production [23]
   Procoagulant effect on platelets [21]
   Impairment of fibrinolysis [24]
   Interference with the thrombomodulin–protein S–protein C pathway [25]
   Induction of procoagulant activity on endothelial cells and/or monocytes [26]
   Disruption of the annexin V cellular shield [13]
   Abnormal cytotrophoblast expression of adhesion molecules in pregnancy [27]

While it is widely accepted that the presence of aPL is associated with thrombosis, the importance of all of the cellular consequences and interactions resulting from aPL is not clearly understood [1,39,41].

The importance of B-2-GP I in binding of aCL as a cofactor is well recognized. However, the mechanisms by which anti–B-2-GP I antibodies bind B-2-GP I are unclear [26]. It appears that B-2-GP I functions as a mild natural inhibitor of contact activation of coagulation [42]. B-2-GP I inhibits platelet function [43,44], down-regulates the activation of Hageman factor [45] and the contact phase of coagulation, prevents the binding of protein S by its

> **Box 3: Unresolved issues in diagnosis**
>
> *Established criteria*
>
> 1999 Sapporo International Consensus Statement on Preliminary Criteria for the Classification of the Antiphospholipid Syndrome [29]
>
> 2006 International Consensus Statement on an Update of the Classification Criteria for Definite Antiphospholipid Syndrome
>
> *Unresolved issues*
>
> Addition of a category for pre-antiphospholipid syndrome [15]
>
> Addition of a category for microangiopathic phospholipid syndrome [15]
>
> Criteria for a "definite" diagnosis amended to eliminate aCL and replace this with anti–B-2-GP I [30]
>
> Addition of IgA to testing for aPL [31,32]
>
> Addition of testing for anti-prothrombin antibodies [30]
>
> Addition of testing for anti–annexin V antibodies in patients with recurrent pregnancy loss [30]
>
> Addition of testing for other aPL
>
> Defining the "best" testing strategy to detect lupus anticoagulant

plasma inhibitor, C4b-binding protein [46], and inhibits tissue factor activity [47]. Interestingly, B-2-GP I deficiency is not associated with predisposition to thrombosis [48]. More recent investigation has implicated other activity of B-2-GP I, including binding of factor XI and inhibition of the factor XI by factor XIIa [40]. It appears that B-2-GP I may colocalize with factor XI and thrombin on the platelet surface and regulate thrombin generation. Rahgozar and colleagues [40] have demonstrated that anti–B-2-GP I antibodies actually potentiate the B-2-GP I–mediated inhibition of factor XI activation by thrombin, thus inhibiting coagulation, rather than inducing thrombosis. This finding, once again, leaves open the question of the pathogenesis of APS and the role of B-2-GP I. Also, because a variety of experimental studies have used systems that do include the presence of B-2-GP I, it is possible that previous studies may have led to erroneous conclusions regarding APS pathogenesis [40].

Just as questions remain regarding the molecular and cellular effects of autoantibodies to aPL and B-2-GP I, the relationship between the activation of intrinsic coagulation and clinical thrombosis remains a subject of investigation. It may be that more than one mechanism is involved and that these are different in patients with different clinical manifestations [39]. Antibodies to a variety of phospholipids and phospholipid-binding proteins now have been recognized, and each may be associated with unique clinical consequences. Although a hallmark of thrombophilia is the propensity for both venous and arterial thrombosis in the same patient, patients with APS tend to have either recurrent arterial or venous events [49]. Arterial thrombosis is primarily driven by platelet

> **Box 4: Unresolved issues in management**
>
> Type of therapy: antiplatelet versus antithrombin agents [33]
>
> The intensity of therapy: target level of international normalized ratio for warfarin therapy [1]
>
> The most accurate method of confirming treatment efficacy: the ratio of prothrombin time (PT) to partial thromboplastin time (PTT) or other laboratory studies [34]
>
> The duration of treatment: no therapy, time-limited therapy versus lifelong therapy [35]
>
> *Optimal management during pregnancy and delivery* [36]
>
> *Optimal management of catastrophic APS* [37]
>
> Anticoagulation
>
> Corticosteroid therapy
>
> Plasma exchange with fresh frozen plasma
>
> Intravenous immune globulin
>
> Rituximab

aggregation while venous thrombosis is driven by activation of the coagulation cascade. aPL procoagulant effects on platelets and endothelial cells may be the mechanisms that trigger arterial events in APS patients. Meanwhile, other mechanisms, such as impairment of fibrinolysis, induction of the expression of tissue factor, and interference with the thrombomodulin–protein S–protein C systems, may be the predominant triggers for venous events in APS patients [39,40]. In addition, it remains unclear why some patients with aPL develop thrombosis and others do not. Furthermore, the triggers for thrombosis in patients with previously asymptomatic aPL are poorly understood.

In considering the pathobiology of APS, it is clear that much remains to be understood. There is debate concerning the triggering events, the molecular mechanisms, and the critical links between pathologic changes at the cellular level and clinical thrombosis. Because these critical questions remain unanswered, precise diagnosis and therapy remain challenging and prognostication for the individual patient continues to be difficult.

DIAGNOSIS

Before the 2006 publication of the International Consensus Statement on an Update of the Classification Criteria for Definite Antiphospholipid Syndrome [50], the diagnosis of "definite" APS was made by following the 1999 Sapporo International Consensus Statement on Preliminary Criteria for the Classification of the Antiphospholipid Syndrome [29]. While the 2006 criteria represent an improvement over the 1999 criteria, a variety of patient subsets still do not fit the strict 2006 criteria, as Asherson [15] has pointed out. The "pre-APS" (probable APS) group includes individuals who have such conditions as livedo reticularis, chorea, thrombocytopenia, fetal loss, and cardiac valve lesions, and who do not fulfill all of the criteria for diagnosis but at a later time develop thrombosis and are then diagnosed with APS. The patients who have microangiopathic phospholipid syndromes include those with thrombotic microangiopathy (thrombotic thrombocytopenic purpura, hemolytic uremic syndrome, HELLP [hemolysis, elevated liver enzyme, and low platelets] syndrome, and catastrophic APS), and patients who have aPL without larger vessel thrombosis [15]. Patients with typical, life-threatening, catastrophic APS may also not fit the strict 2006 International Consensus criteria.

The 2006 International Consensus Statement on an Update of the Classification Criteria for Definite Antiphospholipid Syndrome redefined the diagnostic criteria in light of recent studies. Outstanding issues addressed by the changes from the 1999 to the 2006 criteria include the addition of anti–B-2-GP I antibodies to the laboratory criteria and the more precise definitions regarding the maternal–fetal complications cited among the clinical criteria [50]. Special emphasis is also now given to the other risk factors that may play important roles in the propensity for thrombosis, such as atherosclerotic risk factors and other thrombophilic disorders. Certainly, continuing attention is required to update and possibly modify the criteria for a "definite" diagnosis. A variety of questions remain with respect to diagnosis of APS (see Box 3).

Current Laboratory Criteria for the diagnosis of APS include high titers of aCL or B-2-GP I IgG or IgM antibodies or lupus anticoagulant present on two or more occasions 12 weeks apart [50]. Problems with the laboratory diagnosis of APS remain [28]. Solid phase assays are widely available for the detection and quantification of antibodies to aCL, B-2-GP I, prothrombin, annexin V, and phosphatidylserine, phosphatidylethanolamine, phosphatidylcholine, phosphatidylglycerol, phosphatidylinositol, and phosphatidic acid.

Unfortunately, results vary considerably among laboratories. The First French Anticardiolipin Standardization Workshop found an interlaboratory coefficient of variation for aPL IgG of greater than 70% and a within-run coefficient of variation of 10% [51]. A study by Favoloro and Silvestrini [52] demonstrated an interlaboratory coefficient of variation for aCL IgG and IgM of over 50%. Different laboratories frequently disagreed on whether the aCL were positive or negative. General laboratory standards require interlaboratory consensus of 90% or more in most tests. This is clearly an area of concern in APS testing and the primary basis for requiring repeat testing and agreement on two or more specimens for a "definite" diagnosis [29,50].

The laboratory diagnosis of lupus anticoagulant has proven challenging. The primary coagulation screening study for diagnosis is the activated partial thromboplastin time (aPTT). This phospholipid-based assay becomes prolonged in the presence of a lupus anticoagulant. A mixing study is performed using a 1:1 mix with normal plasma followed by prolonged incubation to determine a correction in aPTT prolongation. In the presence of aPL, the addition of normal plasma and 2 hours or more incubation time will fail to correct the aPTT prolongation. The addition of phospholipid usually corrects the aPTT. Detection of "weak" lupus anticoagulant may be difficult without the use of "platelet poor" normal plasma [28]. The dilute Russell viper venom time (dRVVT) inhibits factor X directly and is not prolonged by the presence of intrinsic factor deficiencies. Prolongation of the dRVVT is more sensitive than the prolongation of the aPTT for detection of lupus anticoagulant [53]. A variety of test systems have been developed to improve diagnostic accuracy. The highest sensitivity and specificity were found with the ratio of dRVVT to dRVVT with high lipid concentration [54]. Because of the many pitfalls in diagnosis, a laboratory decision tree is recommended. Further investigation of a prolonged aPTT is required, with mixing studies, dRVVT, and platelet neutralization procedures. Criteria for the diagnosis of lupus anticoagulant are well established [55] and are included in the 2006 International Consensus Criteria [29,50]. When the diagnosis remains in question, additional testing may be useful. One such test is the hexagonal phase phospholipid neutralization assay [28]. Close correlation between laboratory testing and clinical features is required for accurate diagnosis [56]. Newer approaches to laboratory diagnosis continue to evolve [57].

In patients who present with a history of thrombosis or recurrent miscarriage and who fulfill laboratory criteria for the diagnosis of aPL, there is no controversy regarding the diagnosis. Patients who test positive for aPL and who do not have a history of thrombosis that fits the 2006 International Consensus criteria [29,50] present another challenge. These patients may be tested because of symptoms consistent with pre-APS or microangiopathic phospholipid syndromes, as discussed earlier [15]. Patients may also present with clinical features typical of APS but fail to fulfill the laboratory criteria for a diagnosis of definite APS, or may test positive for aPL but lack clinical criteria for a definite diagnosis. The 2006 criteria addressed many of these patient subsets by specifically defining categories for patients with cardiac valvular disease and aPL, livedo reticularis with aPL, nephropathy with aPL, and thrombocytopenia with aPL. Patients in these groups share clinical features and test positive for aPL, but do not fulfill the 2006 criteria for a definite diagnosis of APS [50].

Because laboratory testing provides less than optimal sensitivity and specificity and is potentially misleading, testing is only indicated in patients suspected of having APS on clinical grounds. Repeat testing is required to make a "definite" diagnosis. Thus, any positive test results should be repeated two or more times 12 weeks apart [50]. Additional confirmatory studies may be indicated in patients with equivocal results, especially in attempting to confirm the suspected diagnosis of lupus anticoagulant. Just as other indices of autoimmunity, the levels of aPL and lupus anticoagulant may vary. Titers may be initially negative and later positive and low titers may become higher or high titers later may become lower [16,58]. There remains no consensus on whether later repeat testing should be performed and whether the results of such repeat studies should affect therapy.

The choice of tests to order in each patient and the interpretation of results remains a matter of considerable study. In patients with definite APS, autoantibodies have been identified to the following:

Anionic phospholipids (eg, aCL and antiphosphatidylserine)
Zwitterionic phospholipids (eg, antiphosphatidylethanolamine)
B-2-GP I
Prothrombin
Thrombin
Annexin V
Antiphosphatidylserine–prothrombin complex
Antithrombin III–thrombin complex
Tissue factor–factor VIIa complex
Protein C
Protein S
Thrombomodulin
Factor XI
Factor XII
High- and low–molecular-weight kininogen
Prekallikrein
Sulphatides
Protein Z–protein Z protease inhibitor system
Tissue plasminogen activator
Plasmin
Platelet-activating factor
Oxidized low-density lipoprotein
High-density lipoprotein
Apolipoprotein A-1
Endothelial cells
Complement component C4
Complement factor H
Antimitochondrial antibody type 5
Malondialdehyde-modified lipoprotein(a) (Table 1) [28,41]

Testing for any of these autoantibodies must be guided by studies demonstrating the clinical utility of the results. It has been accepted that the presence of aCL and lupus anticoagulant is associated with thrombosis. The presence of lupus anticoagulant is a more powerful predictor than the presence of aCL. Multiple studies have confirmed that the presence of high-titer aCL IgG is associated with thrombosis. It is also generally agreed that a similar association exists with IgM antibodies, although the data in this case are less convincing [59]. The inclusion of high-titer IgG and/or IgM and lupus anticoagulant in the 2006 International Consensus criteria are based on these findings [29,50].

The analysis by Galli and colleagues [30] of data from the Warfarin Anti-Phospholipid Syndrome study, published in 2007, seems to contradict prior studies and demonstrates that recurrent thrombosis and miscarriage relates to the presence of autoantibodies to B-2-GP I but not to aCL of any isotype. Accordingly, Galli and colleagues recommend that the criteria for a "definite" diagnosis be

Table 1
Autoantibodies identified in patients with APS and their clinical relevance

Antigen	Clinical application
Anionic phospholipids (eg, anticardiolipin, antiphosphatidylserine)	Antibodies to IgG/IgM in Consensus criteria
Zwitterionic (eg, antiphosphatidylethanolamine)	No guidelines but testing recommended in specific settings
Beta-2-glycoprotein I	Strong correlation with thrombosis
Prothrombin	Emerging application
Annexin V	Correlation with pregnancy loss
Thrombin	None
Antithrombin III–thrombin complex	None
Tissue factor–factor VIIa complex	None
Protein C	None
Protein S	None
Thrombomodulin	None
Factor XI	None
Factor XII	None
High– and low–molecular-weight kininogen	None
Prekallikrein	None
Sulphatides	None
Protein Z–protein Z protease inhibitor system	None
Tissue plasminogen activator	None
Plasmin	None
Platelet-activating factor	None
Oxidized low-density lipoprotein	None
High-density lipoprotein	None
Apolipoprotein A-1	None
Endothelial cells	None
Complement component C4	None
Complement factor H	None
Antimitochondrial antibody type 5	None
Malondialdehyde-modified lipoprotein(a)	None

Data from Ozturk MA, Haznedaroglu IC, Turgut M, et al. Current debates in antiphospholipid syndrome: the acquired antibody-mediated thrombophilia. Clin Appl Thromb Hemost 2004;10(2):89–126; and Mackworth-Young CG. Antiphospholipid syndrome: multiple mechanisms. Clin Exp Immunol 2004;136(3):393–401.

amended to eliminate aCL and to add anti–B-2-GP I. Associations with arterial and venous thrombosis were confirmed for patients with IgG anti–B-2-GP I and anti-prothrombin antibodies. Risk for arterial and total thromboses was especially high for patients with both lupus anticoagulant and anti–B-2-GP I antibodies. Patients positive for lupus anticoagulant who also had B-2-GP I and anti–annexin V antibodies were found to be at risk for recurrent miscarriage and thromboses. Also noted was a strong association between anti–annexin V antibodies and recurrent miscarriage. Antibodies of the IgM isotype to protein S and the lupus ratio of the dilute prothrombin time were associated with future risk for thrombosis. As no other positive IgM antibodies were predictive of future thrombosis or miscarriage, it was noted that measurement of IgM was of little value. The measurement of anti–annexin V antibodies and anti-prothrombin antibodies was recommended in certain situations [30].

Another issue has been whether aCL of the IgA isotype are associated with thrombosis. Some studies have noted an association [60], while others have not [61]. aCL IgA has not been measured routinely and debate continues as to the clinical relevance of an elevated titer [31]. It is not generally recommended that the diagnostic criteria be expanded to include the IgA isotype. However, this remains a topic of debate. Bick [32] have recommended including the measurement of IgA in the laboratory assessment for aCL. The study by Selva and colleagues [62] of 795 patients, however, demonstrated aCL IgA positivity in only 2 patients, both also positive for IgG aCL. The analysis contained in the Miyakis [50] summary of the 2006 criteria notes that testing for IgA is primarily useful for identification of APS subgroups, such as African Americans with systemic lupus erythematosus and patients with connective tissue disease associated with thrombocytopenia, skin ulcers, and cutaneous vasculitis.

Laboratory testing for anti-prothrombin antibodies has not routinely been recommended in the evaluation of patients with suspected thrombophilia. The prevalence of anti-prothrombin antibodies in patients with APS has been reported from 50% to 90% of patients [63]. Some studies have demonstrated an association with thrombosis [64,65] and other studies have not [66]. Analysis of the Warfarin Anti-Phospholipid Syndrome study data suggests a potential role for anti-prothrombin testing [30].

Anti–annexin V is a tissue and circulating phospholipid-binding protein with high affinity for anionic phospholipids and functions as an anticoagulant by displacing coagulation factors from phospholipid surfaces [28]. Autoantibodies to annexin V are reported in a variety of clinical settings, including those involving patients with recurrent thrombosis and miscarriage. In patients with systemic lupus erythematosus, the finding of anti–annexin V IgG antibodies was reported to be associated with a high incidence of arterial or venous thrombosis, prolonged aPTT, and recurrent miscarriage [67]. There has been, however, conflicting data regarding the prognostic value of anti–annexin V antibodies [68]. The data from the Warfarin Anti-Phospholipid Syndrome study provide stronger evidence for the use of anti–annexin V antibodies as a predictor of future thrombosis or miscarriage [30].

There remains a lack of consensus regarding the utility of testing for other anionic and zwitterionic aPL, often referred to as "subtypes." These include phosphatidylserine, phosphatidylethanolamine, phosphatidylcholine, phosphatidylglycerol, phosphatidylinositol, and phosphatidic acid. Studies have demonstrated association with thrombosis for antiphosphatidylserine [69] and antiphosphatidylethanolamine [70]. Some investigators have noted that these "subtypes" may be present in patients without detectable aCL and have advocated testing for them [70,71]. Other investigators have advised that testing for these noncardiolipin phospholipid antibodies is not indicated [72].

The laboratory measurement of autoantibodies in patients with suspected APS remains a subject of research. Review of the literature and clinical practice make it clear that, lacking consensus, a variety of approaches to diagnosis may be used. Generally, a panel of studies is ordered, including the aPTT with mixing study and dRVVT in search of lupus anticoagulant, and IgG, IgM, and possibly IgA assays for aCL. Assessment for B-2-GP I antibodies should be routinely included in the diagnostic panel. In addition, it appears that to this should be added anti–annexin V antibodies, especially in patients with recurrent miscarriage. While broad recommendations are not yet available, it appears that assay for anti-prothrombin antibodies may also soon be included. The inclusion of analysis for other aPL and for other antibodies associated with APS remains controversial and the subject for further investigation.

MANAGEMENT

The management of patients with APS has proven challenging and the subject of numerous studies. Generally, treatment may be divided into the following several categories:

Management of acute large-vessel thrombosis
Management of "pre-APS" (probable APS) and microangiopathic APS
Management of catastrophic APS
Management during pregnancy
Prevention of initial and recurrent thromboses

Bick [32] has divided APS into 6 subgroups. Treatment guidelines have been offered for each group. Well-controlled trials have not, however, verified these recommendations. Many clinical trials support guidelines and expert recommendations. However, in the area of treatment, few large, controlled trials have taken place. Debate and controversy surround the questions of the type of therapy, the intensity of therapy, the most accurate method of confirming treatment efficacy, the duration of treatment, and how best to manage specific clinical circumstances, such as surgery and delivery (see Table 1).

Intervention with anticoagulation is the primary treatment for any patient presenting with acute large-vessel venous or arterial thrombosis. There is a difference, however, between patients with venous versus those with arterial disease. As discussed earlier, in patients with arterial thrombosis, platelet aggregation plays a central role. If the patient has not previously been diagnosed with APS, the mainstay of therapy for arterial thrombosis is usually antiplatelet therapy. The patient with APS, however, requires the addition of anticoagulation therapy with unfractionated or low–molecular-weight heparin followed by warfarin anticoagulation [1]. Patients with acute myocardial infarction and APS have been treated successfully with thrombolytic therapy [73] and also intracoronary stents, followed by anticoagulation [74]. At issue has been how long to treat patients and with what intensity of anticoagulation [75].

Patients with acute stroke, the most common arterial thromboembolic disorder in patients with APS, are managed initially based on clinical criteria. It appears that whether or not the diagnosis of APS is known before presentation with new neurologic symptoms, therapy should be guided by well-established criteria for stroke management. If therapy can be provided within 3 hours of onset and all inclusion criteria are met, thrombolytic therapy may be indicated [76]. There are, however, no large trials of thrombolytic therapy in patients with APS, whether known at the time of the stroke onset or diagnosed at a later time. Post-stroke therapy also remains a subject of investigation and it is not clear what optimum therapy should be [77]. The data from the Antiphospholipid Antibody in Stroke Study Group subset of the Warfarin Versus Aspirin Recurrent Stroke Study demonstrate, contrary to other studies, that there is no difference between aspirin and warfarin in prevention of recurrent stroke [78]. Similar conclusions have been reached in other trials [79,80].

The treatment of acute venous thromboembolism follows well-established guidelines and is independent of the diagnosis of APS [81]. Anticoagulation with low–molecular-weight heparin is favored over unfractionated heparin and should be administered in a full anticoagulation dose. Anticoagulation with warfarin should also be initiated with the dose adjusted to achieve a therapeutic international normalized ratio (INR) of at least 2.0 to 2.9.

Prevention of recurrent thrombosis after acute arterial or venous thrombosis is the subject of considerable investigation and unresolved issues remain. Three retrospective studies have demonstrated that the rate of recurrent thrombosis is reduced by warfarin anticoagulation. In the small series by Derksen and colleagues [82], the recurrence rate at 8 years was 0% for patients anticoagulated and the recurrence rate for patients in whom therapy was stopped was 50% at 2 years and 78% at 8 years. Recurrence also correlates with the intensity of anticoagulation. It has been well established that patients with an INR of less than 1.9 are vulnerable to recurrent thrombosis [49]. The rate of recurrence in patients without optimal anticoagulation is as high as 70% [49,82]. It remains unclear whether high-intensity warfarin therapy is of greater benefit. The report of Crowther and colleagues [83] compared intermediate therapy (2.0 to 3.0) and high-intensity therapy (3.0 to 4.0) in a carefully controlled setting. The benefits and bleeding risks for both treatment groups were essentially the same. Current guidelines recommend intermediate levels of anticoagulation and care to avoid subtherapeutic doses [1]. The appropriate duration of therapy is also unclear. Patients with venous thromboembolism and APS who discontinue therapy have a high risk of recurrence. Therapy, however, is accompanied by a risk of hemorrhage [35]. Patients with venous or arterial thrombotic events and aPL may require lifelong therapy. Monitoring warfarin presents additional challenges as aPL may interfere with the aPTT and prothrombin time test system phospholipid substrate [34].

Aspirin alone may be inadequate to prevent recurrence [33]. Patients with arterial thrombosis and APS may benefit more than patients with venous thrombosis from the addition of antiplatelet therapy. Caution is required, however, in view of the increased risk of hemorrhage associated with such dual therapy. Patients who are not candidates for aspirin therapy may benefit from substitution with clopidogrel [32]. In addition, therapy is complicated by the potential presence of aspirin and/or clopidogrel resistance [36,84].

APS is a proven, treatable cause of recurrent miscarriage. Management of APS in pregnancy presents a variety of challenges and several unanswered questions remain. Because of the significant potential for teratogenic effects from warfarin, anticoagulation during pregnancy requires the use of heparin or low–molecular-weight heparin, rather than warfarin. Full-dose anticoagulation is recommended for patients with a history of venous thromboembolism, but it is unclear if lower doses are adequate in patients with a history of only recurrent pregnancy loss. The addition of aspirin to low-dose heparin or low–molecular-weight heparin in a prophylactic dose has been demonstrated to be highly effective with a successful pregnancy rate as high as 97% [85]. Also unclear is the appropriate time

---

Box 5: Preliminary criteria for the classification of catastrophic APS[a]

1. Evidence of involvement of $\geq$ organs, organ systems, and/or tissues[b]
2. Development of manifestations simultaneously or in <1 week
3. Conformation by histopathology of small-vessel occlusion in at least one organ/tissue[c]
4. Laboratory confirmation of the presence of aPL (lupus anticoagulant and/or aCL and/or anti–B-2-GP I antibodies)[d]

Definite catastrophic APS

All four criteria, except for involvement of only two organs, systems, and/or tissues

Probable catastrophic APS

All four criteria, except for the absence of laboratory confirmation of the presence of aPL at least 6 weeks after a first positive result (due to the early death of a patient never tested for aPL before onset of catastrophic APS)

Possible catastrophic APS

Criteria 1,2, and 4

Criteria 1,3, and 4, plus the development of a third event in >1 week but <1 month, despite anticoagulation treatment

[a]Proposed and accepted during the 10th International Congress on Antiphospholipid Antibodies (aPL), September 2002, in Taormina, Sicily [86].
[b]Clinical evidence of vessel occlusions, confirmed by imaging techniques when appropriate. Renal involvement is defined by a 50% rise in serum creatinine, severe systemic hypertension (>180/100 mm Hg), and/or proteinuria (>500 mg/24h).
[c]Histopathological confirmation requires significant evidence of thrombosis, although vasculitis occasionally may coexist.
[d]If the patient had not been previously diagnosed as having APS, the laboratory confirmation requires detection of the presence of aPL on two or more separate occasions at least 6 weeks apart (not necessarily at the time of the event), as defined in the International Consensus Statement on Preliminary Criteria for the Classification of the Antiphospholipid Syndrome [29].

period for postpartum therapy. As the risk of thrombosis is as high or higher in the postpartum period than in the antepartum period, patients with APS require continued therapy. No properly designed clinical trials are available to guide therapy [1].

Catastrophic APS is characterized by multiple organ dysfunction resulting from widespread microvascular thrombosis. Many questions persist in this difficult group of patients. The criteria for diagnosis are established but are properly identified as "preliminary" (Box 5) [86]. Further investigation is needed to guide diagnosis. Treatment has been studied in limited numbers of patients. Current therapy remains anticoagulation with heparin, accompanied by glucocorticoid therapy and either plasmapheresis or intravenous immune globulin (Box 6) [37]. Alternative treatments have included rituximab, plasma exchange, and the possible addition of cyclophosphamide in patients with systemic lupus erythematosus. Aggressive critical care management of multiple organ dysfunction syndrome is also essential for survival. Because information regarding proper management is from case series and not controlled trials, and because precise understanding of pathogenesis is lacking, many questions remain. The current limited understanding of the syndrome impedes progress to more effective and standardized therapy [87]. Data from the Catastrophic

---

Box 6: Treatment options for catastrophic APS[a]

Standard therapies

Anticoagulation: intravenous heparin followed by lifelong warfarin [37,86,87]

High-dose corticosteroids: methylprednisolone 1–2 mg/kg/d for 3–5 days [37,86,87]

Plasma exchange with or without fresh frozen plasma; fresh frozen plasma especially if schistocytes present [86,87]

Intravenous immune globulin [86,87]

Cyclophosphamide, especially if associated with systemic lupus erythematosus flares [37,86]

Optional therapies

Fibrinolytic therapy [37,86]

Rituximab [87]

Prostacyclin [86]

Ancrod [86]

Defibrotide [86]

Anticytokine treatment [86,87]

[a]Therapeutic guidelines included in the 10th International Congress on Antiphospholipid Antibodies, September 2002, in Taormina, Sicily.

Antiphospholipid Syndrome registry may, in time, provide more reliable treatment guidelines [87].

No one yet has identified the best therapy for patients with "pre-APS" and manifestations of microangiopathic APS [15]. Trials have not addressed the question of whether some type of prophylactic therapy is indicated before a thrombotic event occurs and before the patient truly fulfills the criteria for a "definite" diagnosis according to the 2006 International Consensus Statement [29,50]. Considering the risk of a first thrombotic event in patients with these problematic subsets, some type of antiplatelet or anticoagulation therapy may be indicated. This should be the subject of future investigation [15].

SUMMARY

An overview of the subject of APS provides clear evidence that much remains to be understood. Questions remain regarding the initial triggering events and the pathogenetic mechanisms leading to thrombosis. Limited understanding of pathogenesis has also resulted in considerable uncertainty concerning the use and clinical relevance of laboratory tests for aPL and antiphospholipid binding proteins. The widely accepted 2006 International Consensus Criteria [29] are now challenged in light of recent analysis of trial data, which contradicts earlier studies [30]. Treatment guidelines are not well supported by clinical trial data in many areas of management. Significant debate remains regarding important issues, such as the type, intensity, and duration of anticoagulation therapy. Finally, management of catastrophic APS is based on case series and much more information is needed for the development of strong, evidence-based recommendations.

References

[1] Levine JS, Branch DW, Rauch J. The antiphospholipid syndrome. N Engl J Med 2002;346(10):752–63.
[2] Haserick J, Long R. Systemic lupus erythematosus preceded by false-positive serologic tests for syphillis: presentation of five cases. Ann Intern Med 1952;37:559–65.
[3] Moore J, Mohr C. Biologically false positive tests for syphilis: type, incidence, and cause. JAMA 1952;150:467.
[4] Rand JH. The antiphospholipid syndrome. In: Beutler E, editor. Williams hematology. 6th edition. New York: McGraw-Hill; 2001. p. 1715–33.
[5] Conley C, Hartmann R. A hemorrhagic disorder caused by circulating anticoagulant in patients with disseminated lupus erythemasosus. J Clin Invest 1952;31:621.
[6] Bowie W, Thompson J, Pascuzzi C, et al. Thrombosis in systemic lupus erythematosus despite circulating anticoagulants. J Clin Invest 1963;62:416.
[7] Harris EN, Gharavi A, Boey M, et al. Anticardiolipin antibodies: detection by radioimmunoassay and association with thrombosis in systemic lupus erythematosus. Lancet 1983;2:1211–4.
[8] Hughes G. The anticardiolipin syndrome. Clin Exp Rheumatol 1985;3:285.
[9] Galli M, Comfurius P, Barbui T, et al. Anticoagulant activity of B2-glycoprotein-I is potentiated by a distinct subgroup of anticardiolipin antibodies. Thromb Haemost 1992;68: 297–300.

[10] McNeil H, Simpson R, Chesterman C, et al. Anti-phospholipid antibodies are directed against a complex antigen that includes a lipid-binding inhibitor of coagulation: B2-glycoprotein I (apolipoprotein H). Proc Natl Acad Sci USA 1990;87:4120–4.
[11] Hunt J, McNeil H, Morgan G, et al. A phospholipid-beta 2-glycoprotein I complex is an antigen for anticardiolipin antibodies occurring in autoimmune disease but not with infection. Lupus 1992;1:75–81.
[12] Arvieux J, Roussel B, Jacob MC, et al. Measurement of anti-phospholipid antibodies by ELISA using beta 2-glycoprotein I as an antigen. J Immunol Methods 1991;143:223–9.
[13] Hanly J, Smith S. Anti-beta2-glycoprotein I (GPI) autoantibodies annexin V binding and the anti-phospholipid syndrome. Clin Exp Immunol 2000;120:537.
[14] Bick R, Baker W. Antiphospholipid syndrome and thrombosis. Semin Thromb Hemost 1999;25:333–50.
[15] Asherson RA. New subsets of the antiphospholipid syndrome in 2006: "PRE-APS" (probable APS) and microangiopathic antiphospholipid syndromes ("MAPS"). Autoimmun Rev 2006;6(2):76–80.
[16] Miret C, Cervera R, Reverter JC, et al. Antiphospholipid syndrome without antiphospholipid antibodies at the time of the thrombotic event: transient "seronegative" antiphospholipid syndrome? Clin Exp Rheumatol 1997;15:541.
[17] Arnout J, Vermylen J. Current status and implications of autoimmune antiphospholipid antibodies in relation to thrombotic disease. J Thromb Haemost 2003;1:931.
[18] Gharavi A, Pierangeli S, Harris EN. Origin of antiphospholipid antibodies. Rheum Dis Clin North Am 2001;27:551.
[19] Rauch J, Subang R, D'Agnillo P, et al. Apoptosis and the antiphospholipid syndrome. J Autoimmun 2000;15:231.
[20] Horkko S, Miller E, Dudl E, et al. Antiphospholipid antibodies are directed against epitopes of oxidized phospholipids. Recognition of cardiolipin by monoclonal antibodies to epitopes of oxidized low density lipoprotein. J Clin Invest 1996;98:815.
[21] Walenga J, Michal K, Hoppensteadt D, et al. Vascular damage correlates between heparin-induced thrombocytopenia and the antiphospholipid syndrome. Clin Appl Thromb Hemost 1999;5(Suppl 1):S76.
[22] Hellan M, Kuhnel E, Speiser W, et al. Familial lupus anticoagulant: a case report and review of the literature. Blood Coagul Fibrinolysis 1998;9:195.
[23] Pierangeli S, Gharavi A, Harris EN. Experimental thrombosis and antiphospholipid antibodies: new insights. J Autoimmun 2000;15:241.
[24] Takeuchi R, Atsumi T, Ieko M, et al. Suppressed intrinsic fibrinolytic activity by monoclonal anti-beta-2 glycoprotein I autoantibodies: possible mechanism for thrombosis in patients with antiphospholipid syndrome. Br J Haematol 2002;119:781.
[25] Tsakiris DA, Settas L, PM, et al. Lupus anticoagulant-antiphospholipid antibodies and thrombophilia. Relation to protein C-protein S-thrombomodulin. J Rheumatol 1990;17:785.
[26] Koike T, Bohgaki M, Amengual O, et al. Antiphospholipid antibodies: lessons from the bench. J Autoimmun 2007;28(2–3):129–33.
[27] Di Simone N, Castellani R, Caliandro D, et al. Antiphospholipid antibodies regulate the expression of trophoblast cell adhesion molecules. Fertil Steril 2002;77:805.
[28] Ozturk MA, Haznedaroglu IC, Turgut M, et al. Current debates in antiphospholipid syndrome: the acquired antibody-mediated thrombophilia. Clin Appl Thromb Hemost 2004;10(2):89–126.
[29] Wilson W, Gharavi A, Koike T, et al. International consensus statement on preliminary classification criteria for definite antiphospholipid syndrome: report of an international workshop. Arthritis Rheum 1999;42:1309–11.
[30] Galli M, Borrelli G, Jacobsen EM, et al. Clinical significance of different antiphospholipid antibodies in the WAPS (Warfarin in the Anti-Phospholipid Syndrome) study. Blood 2007;110(4):1178–85.

[31] Carreras LO, Forastiero RR, Martinuzzo M. Which are the best biological markers of the antiphospholipid syndrome? J Autoimmun 2000;15:163.
[32] Bick R. Antiphospholipid thrombosis syndromes. Hematol Oncol Clin North Am 2003;17:115.
[33] Khamashta M, Cuadrado M, Mujic F, et al. The management of thrombosis in the antiphospholipid-antibody syndrome. N Engl J Med 1995;332:993–7.
[34] Moll S, Ortel T. Monitoring warfarin therapy in patients with lupus anticoagulants. Ann Intern Med 1997;127:177–85.
[35] Baker RI. Prevention of recurrent thrombosis in the antiphospholipid antibody syndrome: how long and how high with oral anticoagulant therapy? Med J Aust 2004;180(9):436–7.
[36] Snoep JD, Hovens MM, Eikenboom JC, et al. Association of laboratory-defined aspirin resistance with a higher risk of recurrent cardiovascular events: a systemic review and meta-analysis. Arch Intern Med 2007;167(15):1593–9.
[37] Kitchens C. Thrombotic storm: when thrombosis begets thrombosis. Am J Med 1998;104:381–5.
[38] Rand JH. Molecluar pathogenesis of the antiphospholipid syndrome. Circ Res 2002;90:29.
[39] Gharavi AE, Wilson W, Pierangeli S. The molecular basis of antiphospholipid syndrome. Lupus 2003;12(8):579–83.
[40] Rahgozar S, Yang Q, Giannakopoulos B, et al. Beta2-glycoprotein I binds thrombin via exosite I and exosite II: anti-beta2-glycoprotein I antibodies potentiate the inhibitory effect of beta2-glycoprotein I on thrombin-mediated factor XIa generation. Arthritis Rheum 2007;56(2):605–13.
[41] Mackworth-Young CG. Antiphospholipid syndrome: multiple mechanisms. Clin Exp Immunol 2004;136(3):393–401.
[42] Schousboe I. B2-Glycoprotein I: a plasma inhibitor of the contact activation of the blood coagulation pathway. Blood 1985;66:1086–91.
[43] Nimpf J, Bevers E, Bomans P, et al. Prothrombinase activity of human platelets is inhibited by beta2-glycoprotein-I. Biochim Biophys Acta 1986;884:142.
[44] Nimpf J, Wurm H, Kostner G. Beta 2-glycoprotein-I (apo-H) inhibits the release reaction of human platelets during ADP-induced aggregation. Atherosclerosis 1987;63:109.
[45] Henry M, Everson B, Ratnoff D. Inhibition of the activation of Hageman factor (factor XII) by beta2-glycoprotein I. J Lab Clin Med 1988;111:519.
[46] Merrill J, Zhang H, Shen C, et al. Enhancement of protein S anticoagulant function by beta2-glycoprotein I, a major target antigen of antiphospholipid antibodies: interferes with binding of protein S to its plasma inhibitor, C4b-binding protein. Thromb Haemost 1999;81:748.
[47] Ieko M, Yasokouchi T, Sawada K, et al. The influence of beta2-glycoprotein I on tissue factor activity. Semin Thromb Hemost 1998;24:211.
[48] Bancsi L, van der Linden I, Bertina R. Beta 2 glycoprotein I deficiency and the risk of thrombosis. Thromb Haemost 1992;67:649.
[49] Rosove M, Brewer P. Antiphospholipid thrombosis: clinical course after the first thrombotic event in 70 patients. Ann Intern Med 1992;117:303–8.
[50] Miyakis S. International consensus statement on an update of the classification criteria for definite antiphospholipid syndrome (APS). J Thromb Haemost 2006;4:295–306.
[51] Abuaf N, Meyer O, Laperche S, et al. Conclusions of the first French workshop of standardization of anticardiolipin antibody determination associated with autoimmun pathology. Ann Biol Clin (Paris) 1994;52:365.
[52] Favaloro E, Silvestrini R. Assessing the usefulness of anticardiolipin antibody assays: a cautious approach is suggested by high variation and limited consensus in multilaboratory testing. Am J Clin Pathol 2002;118:548.
[53] Gerbutavicius R, Fareed J, Messmore H, et al. Reference ranges of the dilute tissue thromboplastin inhibition and dilute Russell's viper venom titer tests revisited. Clin Appl Thromb Hemost 2002;8:51.

[54] Ruiz-Irastorza G, Egurbide MV, Ugalde J, et al. High impact of antiphospholipid syndrome on irreversible organ damage and survival of patients with systemic lupus erythematosus. Arch Intern Med 2004;164(1):77–82.
[55] Brandt J, Triplett DA, Alving B, et al. Criteria for the diagnosis of lupus anticoagulants: an update. Thromb Haemost 1995;74:1185–90.
[56] Wasmuth J, Minarro D, Homrighausen A, et al. Phospholipid autoantibodies and the antiphospholipid antibody syndrome: diagnostic accuracy of 23 methods studied by variation in ROC curves with number of clinical manifestations. Clin Chem 2002;48:1004.
[57] Passam F, Krilis S. Laboratory tests for the antiphospholipid syndrome: current concepts. Pathology 2004;36(2):129–38.
[58] Silver RM, Pierangeli S, Edwin SS, et al. Pathogenic antibodies in women with obstetric features of antiphospholipid syndrome who have negative test results for lupus anticoagulant and anticardiolipin antibodies. Obstet Gynecol 1997;176:628.
[59] Galli M, Luciani D, Bertolini G, et al. Lupus anticoagulants are stronger risk factors for thrombosis than anticardiolipin antibodies in the antiphospholipid syndrome: a systematic review of the literature. Blood 2003;101:1827.
[60] Diri E, Cucurull E, Gharavi A, et al. Antiphospholipid (Hughes') syndrome in African-Americans: IgA aCL and abeta2 glycoprotein-I is the most frequent isotype. Lupus 1999;8:263.
[61] Bertolaccini ML, Atsumi T, Escudero Contreras A, et al. The value of IgA antiphospholipid testing for diagnosis of the antiphospholipid (Hughes) syndrome in systemic lupus erythematosus. J Rheumatol 2001;28:2637.
[62] Selva O, Ordi R, Monegal F, et al. Anticardiolipin antibodies-relation with other antiphospholipid antibodies and clinical significance. Thromb Haemost 1998;79:282.
[63] Galli M. Should we include anti-prothrombin antibodies in the screening for the antiphospholipid syndrome? J Autoimmun 2000;15:101.
[64] Nojima J, Kuratsune H, Suehisa E, et al. Anti-prothrombin antibodies combined with lupus anticoagulant activity is an essential risk factor for venous thromboembolism in patients with systemic lupus erythematosus. Br J Haematol 2001;114:647.
[65] Lakos G, Kiss E, Regeczy N, et al. Antiprothrombin and antiannexin V antibodies imply risk of thrombosis in patients with systemic autoimmune disease. J Rheumatol 2000;27:924.
[66] Forastiero RR, Martinuzzo M, Cerrato G, et al. Relationship of anti beta2-glycoprotein I and anti-prothrombin antibodies to thrombosis and pregnancy loss in patients with antiphospholipid antibodies. Thromb Haemost 1997;78:1008.
[67] Kaburaki J, Kuwana M, Yamamoto M, et al. Clinical significance of anti-annexin V antibodies in patients with systemic lupus erythematosus. Am J Hematol 1997;54:209.
[68] Ogawa H, Zhao D, Dlott J, et al. Elevated anti-annexin V antibody levels in antiphospholipid syndrome and their involvement in antiphospholipid antibody specificities. Am J Clin Pathol 2000;114:619.
[69] Branch DW, Rote N, Dostal D, et al. Association of lupus anticoagulant with antibody against phosphatidylserine. Clin Immunol Immunopathol 1987;42:63.
[70] Berard M, Chantome R, Marcelli A, et al. Antiphosphatidylethanolamine antibodies as the only antiphospholipid antibodies. I. Association with thrombosis and vascular cutaneous diseases [see comments]. J Rheumatol 1996;23:1369.
[71] Laroche P, Berard M, Rouquette A, et al. Advantage of using both anionic and zwitterionic phospholipid antigens for the detection of antiphospholipid antibodies. Am J Clin Pathol 1996;106:549.
[72] Branch DW, Silver RM, Pierangeli S, et al. Antiphospholipid antibodies other than lupus anticoagulant and anticardiolipin antibodies in women with recurrent pregnancy loss, fertile controls and antiphospholipid syndrome. Obstet Gynecol 1997;89:549.
[73] Ho Y, Chen M, Wu C, et al. Successful treatment of acute myocardial infarction by thrombolytic therapy in a patient with primary antiphospholipid syndrome. Cardiology 1996;87:354.

[74] Jankowski M, Dudek D, Dubiel J, et al. Successful coronary stent implantation in a patient with primary antiphospholipid syndrome. Blood Coagul Fibrinolysis 1998;9:753.
[75] Derksen R, de Groot P. Do we know which patients with the antiphospholipid syndrome should receive long-term high dose anti-coagulation? J Autoimmun 2000;15:255.
[76] Wardlaw J, del Zoppo G, Yamaguchi T, et al. Thrombolysis for acute ischemic stroke. Cochrane Database Syst Rev 2000(2):CD 000213.
[77] Gatenby PA. Controversies in the antiphospholipid syndrome and stroke. Thromb Res 2004;114(5–6):483–8.
[78] Committee TAW. Antiphospholipid antibodies and subsequent thrombo-occlusive events in patients with ischaemic stroke. JAMA 2004;291:576–84.
[79] Pullicino P, Mohr J, Thompson J, et al, ftW-ARSSG. A comparison of warfarin and aspirin for the prevention of recurrent ischaemic stroke. N Engl J Med 2001;345:1444–51.
[80] Group TEASPiRITES. Oral anticoagulation in patients after cerebral ischaemia of arterial origin and risk of intracranial hemorrhage. Stroke 2003;34:45–7.
[81] Haas S. Treatment of deep venous thrombosis and pulmonary embolism: current recommendations. Med Clin North Am 1998;82:495–510.
[82] Derksen R, de Groot P, Kater L, et al. Patients with antiphospholipid antibodies and venous thrombosis should receive long term anticoagulant treatment. Ann Rheum Dis 1993;52:689–92.
[83] Crowther MA, Ginsberg JS, Julian J, et al. A comparison of two intensities of warfarin for the prevention of recurrent thrombosis in patients with the antiphospholipid antibody syndrome. N Engl J Med 2003;349(12):1133–8.
[84] Fefer P, Hod H, Matetzky S. Clopidogrel resistance—the cardiologist's perspective. Platelets 2007;18(3):175–81.
[85] Bick R. Recurrent miscarriage syndrome due to blood coagulation protein/platelet defects: prevalence, treatment and outcome results. DRW Metroplex Recurrent Miscarriage Syndrome Cooperative Group. Clin Appl Thromb Hemost 2000;6:115.
[86] Asherson RA. Catastrophic antiphospholipid syndrome: international consensus statement on classification criteria and treatment guidelines. Lupus 2003;12:530–4.
[87] Erkan D. Therapeutic and prognostic considerations in catastrophic antiphospholipid syndrome. Autoimmun Rev 2006;6:98–103.

INDEX

A

Anetoderma, in antiphospholipid syndrome, 74–75
Annexin V, role in platelet activation in antiphospholipid syndrome, 3–4
Anti-annexin V antibodies, role in platelet activation in antiphospholipid syndrome, 3–4
Anticardiolipin antibodies, detection of, 27
Antiphospholipid antibodies, 2
    detection of, 27–29
    in various infections, 133–139
    role in neurologic conditions, **93–105**
Antiphospholipid syndrome, 1–172
    autoimmune diseases and, **53–65**
        rheumatoid arthritis, 57
        Sjögren's syndrome, 56–57
        systemic lupus erythematosus, 54–56
        systemic sclerosis, 57–59
        systemic vasculitis other than SLE, 59–60
        treatment of, 60–61
    clinical spectrum of, **33–52**
        arterial thrombosis, 44
        asymptomatic antiphospholipid antibodies, 36–37
        bleeding, 47
        cardiac disorders, 45
        catastrophic, 42–43
        definite, 37–40
        dermatologic disorders, 46
        drug-induced, 41
        gastrointestinal disorders, 46
        hematologic disorders, 47
        in children, 47
        infection-associated, 41
        malignancy-associated, 42
        microangiopathic, 40–41
        miscellaneous manifestations, 47
        neurologic disorders, 45
        obstetrical disorders, 45–46
        prevalence, 36
        probable, 37
        pulmonary manifestations, 46
        renal manifestations, 46
        retinal disorders, 46
        seronegative, 37
        venous thrombosis, 43–44
    controversies and unresolved issues in, **153–172**
        diagnosis, 158–163
        management, 163–167
        pathogenesis, 154–158
    cutaneous manifestations of, **67–77**
        anetoderma, 74–75
        atrophic blanche and livedoid vasculopathy, 69–71
        catastrophic antiphospholipid syndrome, 72–73
        idiopathic livedo reticularis with cerebrovascular accidents (Sneddon's syndrome), 69
        livedo reticularis and racemosa, 67–69
        malignant atrophic papulosis (Degos' disease), 71–72
        papular and plaque occlusive lesions, 73–74
    in infectious disease, **131–143**
        antiphospholipid antibodies in various, 133–139
        catastrophic, 139
        historical background, 131–132
        pathogenic hypothesis, 132–133
    in pregnancy, **107–120**
        recurrent miscarriage syndrome, 107–109
            treatment review, 115–117
            versus other thrombophilias leading to, 109–115
    laboratory evaluation of, **19–32**
        anticardiolipin antibodies, detection of, 27
        antiphospholipid antibodies, detection of, 27–29
        lupus anticoagulants, detection of, 22–27
        summation of International Society on Thrombosis and Haemostasis subcommittee session, 29–30

Note: Page numbers of article titles are in **boldface** type.

Antiphospholipid (*continued*)
  malignancy and, **121–130**
    cancer and hypercoagulability, 121–123
    manifestation, 124–126
    prevalence, 123–124
    prognosis, 126–127
  neurological conditions associated with, **93–105**
    antiphospholipid antibodies, 93–94
    catastrophic, 97
    causes, 97
    classification criteria, 94–95
    clinical presentations, 95–97
    diagnostic tools, 97–98
    epidemiology, 94
    management, 98–99
    pathophysiology, 94
    prognosis, 99–100
  relationship between heparin-induced thrombocytopenia and, **1–18**
  role in cardiovascular disease, **79–94**
    coronary artery disease, 79–83
    intracardiac thrombosis, 86–87
    myocardial involvement, 85–86
    pulmonary hypertension, 87–88
    treatment of cardiovascular disease in, 88–91
    valve abnormalities and peripheral embolization, 83–85
  treatment options for, **145–153**
    antithrombotic regimens for, 148
    clinical presentations, 148–149
    prevalence, 149–152
      arterial thrombosis, 151–152
      venous thrombosis, 151
    subgroups of, 145–147

Antithrombin III, blood coagulation alterations in antiphospholipid syndrome, 4

Antithrombotic regimens, for treatment of antiphospholipid syndrome, 148

Arterial thrombosis, in clinical spectrum of antiphospholipid syndrome, 44

Atrophic blanche, in antiphospholipid syndrome, 69–71

Atrophic papulosis, malignant (Degos' disease), in antiphospholipid syndrome, 71–72

Autoimmune diseases, antiphospholipid syndrome and, **53–65**
  rheumatoid arthritis, 57
  Sjögren's syndrome, 56–57
  systemic lupus erythematosus, 54–56
  systemic sclerosis, 57–59
  systemic vasculitis other than SLE, 59–60
  treatment of, 60–61

B

Bacterial infection, antiphospholipid antibodies in, 137

Beta-2-glycoprotein I, role in platelet activation in antiphospholipid syndrome, 3

Biomarkers, in antiphospholipid syndrome and heparin-induce thrombocytopenia, 10–12
  of endothelial dysfunction, 11
  of hemostatic activation, 10
  of inflammation, 11–12
  of platelet activation, 10
  of thrombin generation, 10

Bleeding, in antiphospholipid syndrome, 47

Blood coagulation, alterations in antiphospholipid syndrome, 4

C

Cancer, antiphospholipid syndrome and, 42, **121–130**
  cancer and hypercoagulability, 121–123
  manifestation, 124–126
  prevalence, 123–124
  prognosis, 126–127

Cardiomyopathy, diffuse, in antiphospholipid syndrome, 85–86

Cardiovascular disease, role of antiphospholipid syndrome in, 45, **79–94**
  coronary artery disease, 79–83
  intracardiac thrombosis, 86–87
  myocardial involvement, 85–86
  pulmonary hypertension, 87–88
  treatment of, 88–91
  valve abnormalities and peripheral embolization, 83–85

Catastrophic antiphospholipid syndrome, 42–43
  cutaneous manifestations of, 72–73
  infectious disease and, 139
  neurologic manifestations of, 97
  treatment options for, 168

Cerebrovascular accidents, idiopathic livedo reticularis with, in antiphospholipid syndrome (Sneddon's syndrome), 69

Children, antiphospholipid syndrome in, 47

Clinical presentation, of antiphospholipid syndrome and heparin-induce

INDEX

thrombocytopenia, commonalities in, 7–8
Clinical spectrum, of antiphospholipid syndrome, **33–52**
    arterial thrombosis, 44
    asymptomatic antiphospholipid antibodies, 36–37
    bleeding, 47
    cardiac disorders, 45
    catastrophic, 42–43
    definite, 37–40
    dermatologic disorders, 46
    drug-induced, 41
    gastrointestinal disorders, 46
    hematologic disorders, 47
    in children, 47
    infection-associated, 41
    malignancy-associated, 42
    microangiopathic, 40–41
    miscellaneous manifestations, 47
    neurologic disorders, 45
    obstetrical disorders, 45–46
    prevalence, 36
    probable, 37
    pulmonary manifestations, 46
    renal manifestations, 46
    retinal disorders, 46
    seronegative, 37
    venous thrombosis, 43–44
Clopidogrel, in treatment of antiphospholipid syndrome, 146–148
Coronary artery disease, in antiphospholipid syndrome, 79–83
    atherosclerosis and antiphospholipid antibodies, 79–81
    bypass graft failure and stent thrombosis, 82–83
    myocardial infarction and antiphospholipid antibodies, 81–82
    role of antiphospholipid antibodies in atherogenesis, 81
    treatment of, 88–90
Coxiella burneti infection, antiphospholipid antibodies in, 138
Cutaneous manifestations, of antiphospholipid syndrome, 46, **67–77**
    anetoderma, 74–75
    atrophic blanche and livedoid vasculopathy, 69–71
    catastrophic antiphospholipid syndrome, 72–73
    idiopathic livedo reticularis with cerebrovascular accidents (Sneddon's syndrome), 69
    livedo reticularis and racemosa, 67–69
    malignant atrophic papulosis (Degos' disease), 71–72
    papular and plaque occlusive lesions, 73–74
Cytomegalovirus infection, antiphospholipid antibodies in, 136

D

Dallas Thrombosis Hemostasis Clinical Center, studies of thrombophilias in women with recurrent miscarriage at, 109–111
Dalteparin (Fragmin), in treatment of antiphospholipid syndrome, 148
Degos' disease, in antiphospholipid syndrome, 71–72
Dermatologic disorders, in antiphospholipid syndrome. *See* Cutaneous manifestations.
Diagnosis, of antiphospholipid syndrome, controversies and unresolved issues in, 158–163
Diastolic dysfunction, in antiphospholipid syndrome, 86
Diffuse cardiomyopathy, in antiphospholipid syndrome, 85–86
Drug-induced antiphospholipid syndrome, 41

E

Embolization, peripheral, in antiphospholipid syndrome, 83–85
Endothelial cells, interference with phospholipids in, in antiphospholipid syndrome, 4–5
    role in platelet activation in antiphospholipid syndrome, 3
Endothelial dysfunction, biomarkers of, in antiphospholipid syndrome and heparin-induce thrombocytopenia, 11
Epstein-Barr virus infection, antiphospholipid antibodies in, 137

F

Fibrinolytic deficit, blood coagulation alterations in antiphospholipid syndrome, 4

G

Gastrointestinal disorders, in antiphospholipid syndrome, 46
Glycoprotein I, beta-2, role in platelet activation in antiphospholipid syndrome, 3

H

Hematologic disorders, in antiphospholipid syndrome, 47
Heparin, in treatment of antiphospholipid syndrome, 145–148
Heparin-induced thrombocytopenia, relationship with antiphospholipid syndrome, **1–18**
Hepatitis C, antiphospholipid antibodies in, 133–135
Human immunodeficiency virus (HIV) infection, antiphospholipid antibodies in, 135–136
Human T-lymphotrophic virus-1 (HTLV-1) infection, antiphospholipid antibodies in, 137
Hypercoagulability, cancer and, 121–123
Hypertension, pulmonary, in antiphospholipid syndrome, 87–88
    treatment of, 91

I

Immune-mediated responses, in antiphospholipid syndrome and heparin-induce thrombocytopenia, 8–10
Infection, antiphospholipid syndrome associated with, 41
Infectious diseases, antiphospholipid syndrome in, **131–143**
    antiphospholipid antibodies in various, 133–139
    catastrophic, 139
    historical background, 131–132
    pathogenic hypothesis, 132–133
Inflammation, biomarkers of, in antiphospholipid syndrome and heparin-induce thrombocytopenia, 11
    up-regulation of, in antiphospholipid syndrome, 5
International Society on Thrombosis and Haemostasis, Summation of subcommittee session in Geneva, Switzerland in 2007, 29–30
Intracardiac thrombosis, in antiphospholipid syndrome, 86–87
    treatment of, 90–91

L

Laboratory evaluation, of antiphospholipid syndrome, **19–32**
    anticardiolipin antibodies, detection of, 27
    antiphospholipid antibodies, detection of, 27–29
    lupus anticoagulants, detection of, 22–27
    summation of International Society on Thrombosis and Haemostasis subcommittee session, 29–30
Leprosy, antiphospholipid antibodies in, 138
Leptospirosis, antiphospholipid antibodies in, 138
Leukocytes, role in platelet activation in antiphospholipid syndrome, 3
Livedo racemosa, in antiphospholipid syndrome, 67–69
Livedo reticularis, in antiphospholipid syndrome, 67–69
    idiopathic, with cerebrovascular accidents (Sneddon's syndrome), 69
Livedoid vasculopathy, in antiphospholipid syndrome, 69–71
Low-molecular-weight heparin, in treatment of antiphospholipid syndrome, 145–148
Lupus anticoagulants, detection of, 22–27
Lupus. *See* Systemic lupus erythematosus (SLE).

M

Malignancy, antiphospholipid syndrome and, 42, **121–130**
    cancer and hypercoagulability, 121–123
    manifestation, 124–126
    prevalence, 123–124
    prognosis, 126–127
Malignant atrophic papulosis (Degos' disease), in antiphospholipid syndrome, 71–72
Management, of antiphospholipid syndrome, controversies and unresolved issues in, 163–167
    See also *underspecific manifestations of antiphospholipid syndrome.*
Microangiopathic antiphospholipid syndrome, 40–41
Miscarriage, recurrent, role of antiphospholipid syndrome in, **107–120**
    recurrent miscarriage syndrome, 107–109
    treatment review, 115–117
    versus other thrombophilias leading to, 109–115
Mycoplasma infection, antiphospholipid antibodies in, 138–139

Myocardial involvement, in antiphospholipid syndrome, 85–86
　　diastolic dysfunction, 86
　　diffuse cardiomyopathy, 85–86

N

Necrosis, cutaneous, in antiphospholipid syndrome, 73–74
Neurologic disorders, in antiphospholipid syndrome, 45
Neurological conditions, role of antiphospholipid antibodies in, **93–105**
　　antiphospholipid antibodies, 93–94
　　catastrophic, 97
　　causes, 97
　　classification criteria, 94–95
　　clinical presentations, 95–97
　　diagnostic tools, 97–98
　　epidemiology, 94
　　management, 98–99
　　pathophysiology, 94
　　prognosis, 99–100

O

Obstetrical disorders, in antiphospholipid syndrome, 45–46
Occlusive lesions, papular and plaque, in antiphospholipid syndrome, 73–74

P

Papular occlusive lesions, in antiphospholipid syndrome, 73–74
Papulosis, malignant atrophic (Degos' disease), in antiphospholipid syndrome, 71–72
Paradoxical embolization, in antiphospholipid syndrome, 85
Parvovirus B_{19} infection, antiphospholipid antibodies in, 136
Patent foramen ovale, in antiphospholipid syndrome, 85
Pathogenesis, of antiphospholipid syndrome, controversies and unresolved issues in, 154–158
Phospholipids, in endothelial cells, interference with in antiphospholipid syndrome, 4–5
Plaque occlusive lesions, in antiphospholipid syndrome, 73–74
Platelet activation, biomarkers of, in antiphospholipid syndrome and heparin-induce thrombocytopenia, 10–11
　in antiphospholipid syndrome, 3–4

Pregnancy, antiphospholipid syndrome in, **107–120**
　　recurrent miscarriage syndrome, 107–109
　　treatment review, 115–117
　　versus other thrombophilias leading to, 109–115
Prevention, of neurologic conditions in patients with elevated antiphospholipid antibodies, 98–99
Protein C, blood coagulation alterations in antiphospholipid syndrome, 4
Protein S, blood coagulation alterations in antiphospholipid syndrome, 4
Pulmonary hypertension, in antiphospholipid syndrome, 87–88
　　treatment of, 91
Pulmonary manifestations, in antiphospholipid syndrome, 46

R

Recurrent miscarriage syndrome, antiphospholipid syndrome in, **107–120**
　　treatment review, 115–117
　　versus other thrombophilias leading to, 109–115
Renal manifestations, in antiphospholipid syndrome, 46
Retinal disorders, in antiphospholipid syndrome, 46
Rheumatoid arthritis, antiphospholipid syndrome and, 57

S

Sclerosis, systemic, antiphospholipid syndrome and, 57–59
Seronegative antiphospholipid syndrome, 37
Sjögren's syndrome, antiphospholipid syndrome and, 56–57
Sneddon's syndrome, in antiphospholipid syndrome, 69
Streptococcal infection, antiphospholipid antibodies in, 138
Systemic lupus erythematosus (SLE), antiphospholipid syndrome and, 54–56
Systemic sclerosis, antiphospholipid syndrome and, 57–59

T

Thrombin generation, biomarkers of, in antiphospholipid syndrome and heparin-induce thrombocytopenia, 10

Thrombocytopenia, heparin-induced, relationship with antiphospholipid syndrome, **1–18**
    antibodies, 5–6
    commonalities with antiphospholipid syndrome, 7–12
        clinical presentation, 7–8
        pathological mechanism, 8–12
    mechanism of thrombosis in, 6–7

Thrombophilias, leading to recurrent miscarriage, 109–111

Thrombosis, in clinical spectrum of antiphospholipid syndrome, 43–44
    arterial, 44
    venous, 43–44
    intracardiac, in antiphospholipid syndrome, 86–87
        treatment of, 90–91
    mechanism of, in antiphospholipid syndrome, 2–5

Tissue factor, blood coagulation alterations in antiphospholipid syndrome, 4

Treatment, of antiphospholipid syndrome, options for, **145–152**
    antithrombotic regimens for, 148
    clinical presentations, 148–149
    controversies and unresolved issues in, 163–167
    prevalence, 149–152
        arterial thrombosis, 151–152
        venous thrombosis, 151
    subgroups of, 145–147

V

Vaculitis, systemic, antiphospholipid syndrome and, 59–60

Valve abnormalities, in antiphospholipid syndrome, 83–85
    association between, 83–84
    patent foramen ovale and, 85
    pathogenesis of, 84
    thromboembolic events in, 84–85
    treatment of, 90

Varicella virus infection, antiphospholipid antibodies in, 136–137

Venous thrombosis, in clinical spectrum of antiphospholipid syndrome, 43–44

Moving?

Make sure your subscription moves with you!

To notify us of your new address, find your **Clinics Account Number** (located on your mailing label above your name), and contact customer service at:

E-mail: elspcs@elsevier.com

800-654-2452 (subscribers in the U.S. & Canada)
407-345-4000 (subscribers outside of the U.S. & Canada)

Fax number: 407-363-9661

Elsevier Periodicals Customer Service
6277 Sea Harbor Drive
Orlando, FL 32887-4800

*To ensure uninterrupted delivery of your subscription, please notify us at least 4 weeks in advance of move.